Autism in Pediatric Practice

A CLINICIAN'S GUIDE

Polly J. Panitz, MD

American Academy of Pediatrics
DEDICATED TO THE HEALTH OF ALL CHILDREN®

American Academy of Pediatrics Publishing Staff
Mark Grimes, *Vice President, Publishing*
Jeff Mahony, *Senior Director, Professional and Consumer Publishing*
Sara Weissenborn, *Editor, Professional/Clinical Publishing*
Annika Hawkinson, *Editorial Assistant*
Leesa Levin-Doroba, *Production Manager, Practice Management*
Amanda Helmholz, *Medical Copy Editor*
Soraya Alem, *Manager, Digital Publishing*
Mary Louise Carr, MBA, *Marketing Manager, Professional Resources*

Published by the American Academy of Pediatrics
345 Park Blvd
Itasca, IL 60143
630/626-6000
www.aap.org

The American Academy of Pediatrics is an organization of 67,000 primary care pediatricians, pediatric medical subspecialists, and pediatric surgical specialists dedicated to the health, safety, and well-being of all infants, children, adolescents, and young adults.

While every effort has been made to ensure the accuracy of this publication, the American Academy of Pediatrics does not guarantee that it is accurate, complete, or without error.

The recommendations in this publication do not indicate an exclusive course of treatment or serve as a standard of medical care. Variations, taking into account individual circumstances, may be appropriate.

Statements and opinions expressed are those of the authors and not necessarily those of the American Academy of Pediatrics.

Any websites, brand names, products, or manufacturers are mentioned for informational and identification purposes only and do not imply an endorsement by the American Academy of Pediatrics (AAP). The AAP is not responsible for the content of external resources. Information was current at the time of publication.

The publishers have made every effort to trace the copyright holders for borrowed materials. If they have inadvertently overlooked any, they will be pleased to make the necessary arrangements at the first opportunity.

This publication has been developed by the American Academy of Pediatrics. The contributors are expert authorities in the field of pediatrics. No commercial involvement of any kind has been solicited or accepted in the development of the content of this publication. Financial and conflict of interest disclosures for the author of this book can be found at https://publications.aap.org/aapbooks/pages/ma1223.

Every effort has been made to ensure that the drug selection and dosages set forth in this publication are in accordance with the current recommendations and practice at the time of publication. It is the responsibility of the health care professional to check the package insert of each drug for any change in indications or dosage and for added warnings and precautions.

Every effort is made to keep *Autism in Pediatric Practice: A Clinician's Guide* consistent with the most recent advice and information available from the American Academy of Pediatrics.

Please visit www.aap.org/errata for an up-to-date list of any applicable errata for this publication.

Special discounts are available for bulk purchases of this publication. Email Special Sales at nationalaccounts@aap.org for more information.

Printed in the United States of America

9-534 1 2 3 4 5 6 7 8 9 10
MA1223
ISBN: 978-1-61002-883-7
eBook: 978-1-61002-884-4

Cover and publication design by Linda Diamond

Library of Congress Control Number: 2025947141

American Academy of Pediatrics Reviewers

Committee on Drugs

Committee on Nutrition

Committee on Practice and Ambulatory Medicine

Council on Children With Disabilities

Council on Clinical Information Technology

Council on Genetics

Council on School Health

Section on Administration and Practice Management

Section on Clinical Pharmacology and Therapeutics

Section on Developmental and Behavioral Pediatrics

Section on Neurology

Section on Obesity

Contents

Introduction

The landscape of primary care pediatrics is changing quickly. Pediatric primary care clinicians' traditional roles of providing anticipatory guidance and preventing and treating infectious diseases have evolved, and there is an increased need for pediatric clinicians to participate in the management of the behavioral and developmental health of the children they serve. Today, the pediatric clinician performs developmental surveillance and screening for behavioral and developmental disorders and spends an increasing proportion of their time addressing these pediatric needs. The average pediatric clinician spends as much as 25% of their clinical time addressing behavioral health and school concerns. Concern for possible autism is often raised by families and requires a prompt and thoughtful response from the clinician.

Of 8-year-old children, 1 in 31 is now identified as meeting diagnostic criteria for autism, yet many specialty clinics and professionals evaluating these children have long wait lists, leaving the responsibility for care to the pediatric primary care clinician. Many pediatric clinicians have not received adequate training to address these needs and, as a result, may have varying levels of expertise in developmental disabilities and family-focused care. In addition, clinicians have many competing demands that may affect their ability to provide the services necessary to meet this growing need.

Despite these challenges, the primary care clinician is the one medical specialist who develops trusting long-term relationships with families and has the advantage of following a child over their developmental trajectory. The relationship that evolves between a clinician and the family has tremendous therapeutic value and enables the primary care clinician to monitor progress in the autistic child, identify new challenges as they manifest, and support the family as they prioritize treatment goals and engage with appropriate community resources over the child's lifetime. For these reasons, it is critical that the primary care clinician take an active role in care management for the autistic child.

The pediatric primary care clinician has the opportunity to set the precedent for a strength-based approach to the care of a child on the autism spectrum. Every child has a myriad of strengths, whether they are cognitive assets, specific talents, a compelling smile, a loving nature, or keen interests. Emphasizing and celebrating these strengths while following the child over the lifespan models an approach full of compassion, appreciation, and optimism for all children, especially those with developmental challenges. It is important to assume that all children have cognitive strengths, regardless of their speaking ability, and they should be provided opportunities for educational, social, and vocational engagement. Each child will evolve along their own developmental trajectory, and guiding parents to accept this reality is helpful. Proceeding from this foundation, a clinician models an approach based on hope and optimism. A thorough understanding of the challenges and the therapeutic options available to youth on the spectrum will allow the pediatric primary care clinician to support families as they advocate for their children. The pediatric primary care clinician is not expected to be an autism specialist or to assume responsibility for all the needs of families of children on the spectrum but is encouraged to find opportunities to take on incrementally more responsibility for management of the complexities of their care.

It is my hope that *Autism in Pediatric Practice: A Clinician's Guide* will serve as an educational tool and a practical guide for care of the autistic child that enables clinicians within the medical home to lean into the role of patient care and coordination for families affected by autism. Not only is each child on the spectrum different, but each clinician's expertise is different. This guide can be used to strengthen the clinician's knowledge base and to provide a framework for caring for the autistic child along with practical clinical tools to assist in the primary care setting. This book is meant to serve as a reference for the clinician taking on more responsibilities in chronic care management. The expectation is that the clinician will grow in this role but not be expected to achieve the same scope of care as a specialist.

Although it is advised that the chapters be read in the sequence in which they are presented, this book can also be used as a topical reference as the clinician develops new areas of expertise in autism care. Concepts are presented using hypothetical, fictitious case vignettes that are likely to occur in clinical practice. The teaching points are then discussed in detail in the chapters. A variety of useful tools for screening and documentation are included within the chapters and the Appendixes to aid clinicians in applying the professional practice guidelines in the primary care setting. Relevant parent education handouts and resources are included to augment the care provided.

One of the primary objectives discussed in this book is the early provision of appropriate supports and information that is relevant to the child identified as having developmental features of autism. This book will, as a result, focus on early childhood. There are components in each chapter that address the issues relevant to later childhood, but the predominant focus is providing care for the child and family in early childhood as a diagnosis manifests and evolves. This book seeks to support the practice of the primary care clinician; thus, the term *pediatric primary care clinician* is used often. This term is meant to be inclusive of all those who provide services in the primary care setting: pediatricians, family practitioners, physician assistants, nurse practitioners, and all nurses and trainees. The tools and materials may be relevant to developmental pediatricians or psychiatrists establishing their practice as well.

This book aims to use language that respectfully reflects the diverse preferences within autism communities, alternating between identity-first language (eg, *the autistic child*) and person-first language (eg, *the child on the autism spectrum/on the spectrum*), while reserving the full term, *autism spectrum disorder,* for references to the *Diagnostic and Statistical Manual of Mental Disorders* diagnostic criteria. The terms *parent* and *family* are used regularly to refer to the adults who care for the child. In some cases, this might be grandparents or other adults who have become the child's primary caregiver.

The advice in this guide is an amalgamation of what is available through the research literature, published practice parameters, and prioritized advice from the clinical experience of a community-based developmental pediatrician. The advice will focus on practices that can and should be incorporated into primary care. The hope is that the guidance provided will support the busy primary care clinician as they partner with families to make clinical decisions that will optimize the emotional, physical, and developmental outcomes of children on the spectrum.

Polly J. Panitz, MD

American Academy of Pediatrics Resources

Bridgemohan C, Kaufman B, Johnson DM, Shulman LH, Zuckerman KE, eds. *Caring for Children With Autism Spectrum Disorder: A Practical Resource Toolkit for Clinicians.* 3rd ed. American Academy of Pediatrics; 2020. Accessed December 16, 2025. https://publications.aap.org/toolkits/pages/Autism-Toolkit

Hyman SL, Levy SE, Myers SM, et al; American Academy of Pediatrics Council on Children With Disabilities and Section on Developmental and Behavioral Pediatrics. Identification, evaluation, and management of children with autism spectrum disorder. *Pediatrics.* 2020;145(1):e20193447 PMID: 31843864 doi: 10.1542/peds.2019-3447

CHAPTER

1

Caring for the Autistic Child in the Medical Home

CASE VIGNETTE

Alex is a 4-year-old child who was identified as autistic at age 2 years. His parents have chosen a pediatric practice that prioritizes care coordination and child-centered care. He has most of his appointments with the same clinician, and at each health supervision visit, the primary care clinician incorporates time to sit down face-to-face with the parents to review Alex's progress, mark new accomplishments, and elicit the parents' views on their child's progress. The primary care clinician has reviewed the progress reports from Alex's private therapists and specialists and has a clear understanding of the care goals and recommendations as well as the ways to support and include the family in Alex's therapy. Alex's developmental course is reviewed, and a discussion of care goals, modalities, and resources is offered to the family. After each visit, the parents feel supported, encouraged, and more confident in caring for their child. They report not only on the partnership that has developed with this practice but on the positive effect this has had on their family.

Pediatric primary care clinicians gain a valuable long-term perspective on a child's development through their ongoing relationship with the family. This relationship, strengthened by collaboration with specialists and allied health professionals, fosters a foundation of trust that is essential for effective care. Trust encourages parents and caregivers to share concerns openly, recognize their child's strengths and needs, and seek guidance in addressing developmental challenges. Ideally, families establish care with a pediatric practice in the child's infancy, ensuring that this collaborative and supportive approach begins at the earliest stages of development.

The clinician should prioritize time to listen to and guide the family as they navigate a child's life with autism. The pediatric primary care clinician will need to have a clear understanding of the child's developmental challenges, if any have arisen, and the educational and therapeutic strategies that are being used to address these challenges. To gain this understanding, it can be helpful for the clinician to obtain copies of and review progress reports from the school, private therapists, and specialists who work with the child. The primary care clinician will be the only professional to have both a longitudinal knowledge of the child and a global understanding of the child's care plan. In this way, the pediatric primary care clinician should work toward playing the critical and valuable role of case manager and coordinator of the care the child receives.

The pediatric primary care clinician should have a knowledge base pertinent to autism and its co-occurring conditions. This book aims to provide a systematic approach for monitoring the child's development across domains as well as a selection of autism-specific anticipatory guidance. It also provides the primary care clinician with information on available supports and services and how the clinician can best guide parents through the complicated process of selecting specialists and allied health professionals, prioritizing care goals, and monitoring progress throughout the child's lifetime. To best care for the autistic child, the primary care clinician is encouraged to integrate autism-specific care into the child's routine pediatric care while developing a systematic approach for chronic care management.

Autism is not a static condition and there is no "one size fits all" approach to appropriate supports and services. Ongoing care requires an understanding of the individual child, a knowledge base of autism and development, and an understanding of the need for collaboration with families.

Partnering With Families

The therapeutic value of the partnership between a family and the pediatric primary care clinician cannot be overstated. Children with specific developmental differences and diagnoses may be seen by specialists. Specialist practices are in high demand, have limited availability compared to primary care practices, and may not be a feasible option for some families because accessibility or insurance coverage is narrow or difficult to obtain. The primary care clinician's ability to assume some of the chronic care management of children with developmental concerns and diagnoses is immensely helpful. The resultant positive effect on the family and the deepening of the clinician-parent relationship are likely to provide fulfillment for the clinician in addition to the family. The primary care clinician should prioritize opportunities to foster partnership with parents. Encouraging parents to sit down and share their concerns within pediatric visits is the first step toward providing successful care that addresses the priorities of the family. Later, as the child matures, this partnership will include the child as well.

The **HELP** acronym has been developed by the American Academy of Pediatrics to teach practitioners the elements of effective communication that, among other things, lead to the development of relationships with parents (**Box 1.1**). Using the HELP acronym as a protocol, primary care clinicians can build skills that strengthen their rapport with families and enable effective collaboration as families navigate the many decisions involved in raising a child on the autism spectrum.

BOX 1.1 HELP Acronym

- **H** = **Hope. Hope** facilitates coping by using a strength-based approach to autism.
- **E** = **Empathy. Empathy** is communicated by listening to, acknowledging, and affirming struggles and successes.
- **L** = **Language, Loyalty.** Use the **language** the family uses to restate the struggles, and communicate **loyalty** to and support for the family.
- **P** = **Partner, Permission, Plan. Partner** with the family to identify barriers and goals for care. Ask **permission** to work together on developing a **plan** to meet goals.

Adapted from Foy JM, Green CM, Earls MF; American Academy of Pediatrics Committee on Psychosocial Aspects of Child and Family Health and Mental Health Leadership Work Group. Mental health competencies for pediatric practice. *Pediatrics.* 2019;144(5):e20192757.

When the HELP acronym is used as a protocol for promoting partnership, the first component is creating the opportunity for using active listening skills. Clinicians can allot time for engagement with the child and family at all visits. The pediatric primary care clinician may communicate observations of the child's strengths as these become apparent to help instill a sense of **hope** and optimism. These might include recent skill acquisitions or areas of strength, the clinician keeping in mind that each child will have a unique developmental trajectory. By affirming and acknowledging parents' viewpoints, the clinician may communicate a message of **empathy** that helps solidify the therapeutic relationship. Restating what the parent has shared by using their own **language** assures them that the clinician understands and can address their perspective. The primary care clinician must ask **permission** of the family to enter this type of **partner**ship as they work to identify barriers to progress, goals for care, and strategies for achieving these goals. The primary care clinician should strive to ensure that the family leaves each visit with a **plan** to promote constructive change. This might take the form of parent education and resources, referrals for therapy, new care goals, or guidance on next steps for further assessment.

Validating Parent Concerns and Observations

The developmental concerns of parents have high predictive value and should be validated by the pediatric primary care clinician. Even though 85% of parents of children who subsequently received a diagnosis of autism raised concerns about their child's development in the first 2 years after birth, the average age of diagnosis is older than 4 years. Children and families from groups that have been historically excluded or those living in poverty are more likely to face barriers to accessing care, experience bias within health care settings, and receive diagnoses later as a result.

The clinician should respond to concerns raised by parents, and by any educator or clinician working with the child, at all visits, even in the face of low-likelihood screening results. This approach sets the precedent for future sharing and trust as the clinician-parent relationship strengthens over time. It will increase the clinician's success at the early identification of children with developmental disability and will likely improve long-term outcomes as decisions are made with families about referrals and support.

The pediatric clinician should be sensitive to the language that is used to explain autism. The medical model, on which the *Diagnostic and Statistical Manual of Mental Disorders* criteria are based, views autism as a medical disorder defined by deficits that require change and treatment. On the other hand, many parents and autistic individuals view autism as a variant of naturally occurring abilities and prefer to accept the developmental trajectory of the child while focusing on adapting the child's environment to support their optimal progress. Regardless of which model the professional espouses, the therapeutic value of finding ways to adapt the environment in support of the child's path is an effective approach and should be integrated into the child's care plan. Many individuals view their autism as a part of their identity and prefer to use identity-first language, in which they refer to themselves as an *autistic individual.* Others prefer the use of person-first descriptions, such as the *individual on the autism spectrum/on the spectrum.* It is important that the clinician be sensitive to these differences and support the family and individual's language preferences. The sensitivity to the connotations associated with these terms is important, as is the perspective that autism is an extremely heterogenous entity in which children will have variable developmental trajectories requiring different levels of support and care.

Supporting Understanding and Acceptance

Clinical experience bears out that when a family understands their child's autism diagnosis and its lifelong implications, they observe their child in a more accommodating light. When parents are able to identify their child's strengths as well as the areas of concern, they are more able to accept the trajectory that their child follows as being different from what they expected. In this process, parents are more likely to understand that a child may need comprehensive services and accommodations to support their well-being. The pediatric primary care clinician plays an important role in listening to parents' concerns and providing information that will support this process of understanding the benefit of therapeutic strategies.

The clinician should remain vigilant to how the family responds to receiving a diagnosis without making assumptions about their responses. Fear, grief, confusion, and misunderstanding of a diagnosis may be present when a family first receives an autism diagnosis for their child. Some families may withhold the diagnosis from friends, family, and schools. They may believe that their child will "outgrow" their challenges and may therefore not see the need for support. They may convince themselves that a clinician made an invalid assessment and diagnosis. Children on the autism spectrum are as beautiful and healthy as any child, and it can be challenging for parents to accept a diagnosis that has lifelong implications. Some parents may struggle to accept that their child is on the spectrum because there are preconceived notions, cultural beliefs, or stereotypes of what autism is. Many parents observe cognitive strengths in their child and do not understand how autism could be possible. Others will view their child as having abilities that represent a difference that occurs naturally across a neurodiverse population. The pediatric primary care clinician can help impart or validate the knowledge that each person on the spectrum is different and has their own unique strength profile.

Families benefit from sharing their questions and concerns when learning to understand the significance and potential implications of an autism diagnosis for their child. They seek guidance from the clinician with whom they already have a trusting relationship. The more information about the child and care options that is shared while the parent's concerns are identified and addressed, the more accurate the parent's understanding of their child's strengths, disabilities, and support needs will be. Parents rely on the pediatric primary care clinician to provide information that helps guide their family's decisions about potential supports and services. The foundation the primary care clinician has created with the family enhances their understanding of recommendations made. This is particularly helpful when parents seek feedback about experimental or unsubstantiated interventions that they encounter from other sources.

Unless the clinician has created the opportunity for families to share their questions, concerns, and beliefs, they may find that families feel overwhelmed and unsupported in taking recommended next steps. By providing professional insights, the pediatric clinician can play an integral role in educating and supporting families about autism while working over a lifetime to help families navigate services that support their child and family's unique needs.

Engaging in Care Planning

When parents become overwhelmed by navigating services and supports, they may turn to the pediatric primary care clinician for guidance. Parents must navigate long wait lists and the logistics of insurance reimbursement, and they must rearrange their family's lives and priorities while working out the pragmatics of a care plan. This process can be very stressful, and parents may experience feelings of self-doubt and inadequacy. Many parents initially struggle to successfully engage their children using strategies that may at first seem unfamiliar, unnatural, and time consuming. There is a myriad of overwhelming choices to make, and parents may feel an urgency to make the best decision as soon as possible. Many are influenced by what they read online or on social media sites. They may feel the necessity to ensure that their child is able to "catch up" during the critical years of early childhood. The pediatric clinician plays an important role in reassuring and helping guide the parent in sorting through recommendations from many sources as, together, they assemble a care plan that works to support the child and the family.

The primary care clinician can support parents as they make difficult choices about how to prioritize time and resources. Parents might seek guidance on whether to search for behavioral therapists, seek the involvement of a speech therapist, or rely on their school system's programming. They are faced with decisions about which specialists and allied health professionals are best and which model of care is appropriate. Families will be most comfortable working with therapists who value and incorporate their needs and belief systems. They will need to learn to understand insurance terms such as *in-network* and *out-of-network* coverage and how to determine which therapies their insurance plans will cover. They will need to learn how to navigate wait lists and resources in their communities, including state public assistance and disability service programs, and may rely on the pediatric practice to provide assistance in this process.

The challenges that may arise from the child's developmental course and competing everyday activities can easily tax a family and lead to tremendous amounts of stress. Parents may struggle to balance the needs of their child on the spectrum with those of the family. The black hole of advice and promises for a "cure" found on the internet and parent chat spaces can create overwhelming amounts of guilt for parents who may already be struggling to simply engage their child in a constructive manner. Many will doubt their own judgment and accept therapies that are not helpful or, even worse, that may have negative effects. The opportunity to review these stresses and concerns with a professional who can acknowledge their struggles and offer words of hope, empathy, and encouragement is invaluable. Within this context, the clinician can help families find a pathway that supports the individual child and family.

The pediatric primary care clinician can introduce a stepwise approach to guiding support. As they assist the family in identifying and prioritizing care goals, they can discuss the array of supports and services available. Suggestions should always integrate the options available through early intervention services while referring for private services when possible and indicated. Some types of private services (ie, speech and occupational therapy) might be available more immediately, and others (eg, applied behavior analysis) might have longer wait lists and intake procedures. The primary care clinician can help identify nonmedical care navigators within their practice or community to assist families with this process, and families can be instructed to request the assignment of a case manager through their insurance company or state disability program to further assist them. Referrals for assistance through nonprofit organizations and parent-run groups can be invaluable. The pediatric primary care clinician can be immensely helpful because they are available to listen, support, and guide the family as they devise a road map for the future. Clinicians can support families in this process in the following ways:

- Consider a stepwise approach to referrals: include services more immediately available or of highest priority to the family while they are waiting for other services or those with wait lists and long intake procedures.
- Identify care navigators with lived experience to assist families.
- Request a case manager through the family's insurance provider.
- Identify nonprofit and publicly funded organizations to assist the family.
- Identify parent groups in the community.

Integrating Autism Care With Medical Care

Children who receive a diagnosis of autism are at risk for a complex web of developmental, behavioral, and medical health conditions that require detection, monitoring, and intervention. As a result, they experience an increased need for medical care while facing a paucity of accessible specialty services. Families from populations with access to fewer resources encounter disproportionate barriers to care, including, but not limited to, financial, cultural, and language barriers. Poor access to care and resultant unidentified co-occurring conditions further contribute to poor outcomes and quality of life for these children and their families. The pediatric primary care clinician who will take on responsibility for identification and management of evolving medical and behavioral health conditions at each visit can have a tremendous positive effect on the lives of children and their families. The bulk of this guide is dedicated to this process.

This guide reviews the current medical knowledge about autism, provides tools for screening, defines how the diagnosis is made, and dedicates the bulk of the material to the role of the pediatric primary care clinician in the medical evaluation, identification, and care of the conditions that are known to be more common in those on the spectrum. A review of behavioral management specific to autism and an overview of the special education process are included to encourage the primary care clinician to support parents as they advocate within this process. This guide also provides resources for the primary care clinician that can be used to make each visit more efficient and effective while supporting the process of parent education. Appendix A, Autism Monitoring Tool for the Pediatric Primary Care Clinician, provides a checklist to be used to monitor the progress of the autistic child and provide prompts for the information required at all visits. The information obtained from these screenings for both core features of autism and coexisting medical conditions will help inform care planning at each step. Additionally, Appendix B, Parent Handout: What Is Autism and How Do I Know if My Preschool-Aged Child Is on the Spectrum? is a handout for parents explaining autism and its early clinical signs and includes suggestions to promote engagement.

Promoting Preventive Care

Children on the autism spectrum are less likely to be seen for health supervision visits than are children not on the spectrum. This fact most likely explains why children on the spectrum are less likely to be vaccinated and have fewer opportunities to receive preventive care, such as anticipatory guidance and health surveillance. Despite the lack of credible evidence to support a link between any vaccine and the occurrence of autism in children, some parents are reluctant to have their children vaccinated. Creating the opportunity for parents to voice these concerns is an imperative first step in counseling about vaccines. Some fear that further vaccination will exacerbate the challenges for children who have already received a diagnosis of autism, or they may have concern for causing autism in a sibling. Parents' decisions about vaccinations and health surveillance must be addressed to minimize further health risks. Children on the spectrum are already at risk for poor health outcomes caused by associated medical complexities, poor access to care, medical bias, and financial and cultural barriers that exist in the medical system. For many on the spectrum, the medical visit causes tremendous anxiety and requires significant accommodations to ensure the success of the examination and necessary screening and procedures while minimizing the trauma to the child.

The pattern of not participating in health supervision for children on the spectrum contrasts with the experience of children with other medical conditions that similarly place them at high risk for poor health outcomes. In other high-risk situations, parents are typically more likely to seek the advice of pediatric clinicians and remain diligent in scheduling these visits. The health supervision visit is an opportunity for a primary care clinician to monitor a child's progress, identify coexisting conditions, and engage in care guidance and coordination. These visits also allow families to find the guidance they need to refine care goals and identify appropriate evidence-based supports and services as the child matures.

Creating Opportunities for Autism Care

To meet the needs of families, the pediatric primary care clinician should incorporate protocols for scheduling, preparing, and billing for visits that support the opportunity to address autism-related concerns and should communicate to families that this is a priority. This is discussed in detail in Chapter 4, The Pragmatics of the Pediatric Visit. Research surveys indicate that pediatric primary care clinicians who prioritize and address family concerns and create opportunities for care management achieve a greater level of satisfaction in and collaboration with the family.

Surveys have identified that primary care clinicians are more likely to report a knowledge deficit, lack of time, and low insurance reimbursement as barriers to their ability to meet the needs of their patients on the autism spectrum. Parents may have the expectation that discussion of concerns around their child's autism is irrelevant to the pediatric visit. Expressing an interest in issues specific to the child's autism and creating opportunities for discussion of these issues within each pediatric visit has tremendous value to the child and family. This is exemplified by the case vignette of Alex presented at the beginning of this chapter. Parents may not know that the pediatric visit can be used to review issues related to their child's developmental disability. The remainder of this guide demonstrates an approach to autism care that is relevant to the primary care practice setting.

Ensuring Care Coordination

The pediatric clinician has an understanding of the whole child as they exist along a developmental trajectory within a family unit, a community or culture, and an educational setting. At times, recommendations made by different specialists involved with the child may be conflicting or confusing. It is the pediatric primary care clinician who may have more experience with the child and family to understand these inconsistencies. Coordination across settings can be problematic. For example, a special education instructor might introduce a different communication system or specific communication goal than a private therapist. Different approaches can augment care, but they should not conflict with each other or cause confusion. The school team should coordinate their goals and methodologies for achieving each goal with those recommended by the private therapists and those prioritized by the family. The pediatric clinician is ideally suited to introduce the idea of coordinated care and support across settings and should make an effort to

- Obtain reports and care plans from therapists/educators to coordinate and define goals across settings.
- Create a system for documenting therapies, goals, and progress within the electronic health record that can serve as a care plan.
- Insist on a family-centered approach to support through which the family's goals are included and prioritized.
- Ensure there is an effective parent education component to all therapies.
- Assess for relevant health issues at each visit.
- Facilitate transitions between settings (eg, preschool to elementary school, secondary school to postsecondary education or the community).

Approaching Behavioral Challenges

It is tempting to attribute behavioral challenges to the diagnosis of autism and therefore miss opportunities for better understanding of the needs of the child. This guiding principle is emphasized as each element of care for the child is discussed throughout this guide. Behavioral manifestations often grow out of the child's struggles to meet expectations in a given situation, and they help pinpoint underlying underdeveloped skill sets that suggest the need for supportive strategies. It is important not to make assumptions about behavior or jump to conclusions about the source of the behavior without a careful analysis of causation. A child might present with behavioral challenges not because they have a specific diagnosis but more likely because their communication delay, their sensory vulnerabilities, their constipation, their sleep disruption, or their struggles with flexibility in a dynamic situation result in distress and anxiety. These responses affect their everyday performance, resilience, and adaptability. While there may be a role for medication, especially when there are coexisting conditions, the focus must first be on searching to understand the function or the why of the behavior. The pediatric primary care clinician is pivotal in examining behavioral challenges within a broader context of the child's developmental challenges, coexisting conditions, family and cultural expectations, community factors, and social drivers of health. The pediatric clinician is often the first professional to whom a parent turns as behavioral manifestations of autism evolve. Many behavioral manifestations of autism are very similar to those observed in neurotypical children, but they may present in an atypically persistent, intrusive, and repetitive manner that could interfere with the child's ability to follow requests and engage in social settings. In addition, behavioral manifestations exhibited by the child may be an expression of a medical condition or pain requiring intervention. In this guide, we discuss the need for the clinician to assess presenting behavioral challenges to understand why they occur and how they influence the care of an autistic child. This is addressed more thoroughly in Chapter 9, Autism and Behavioral Challenges: Why They Occur and How to Approach Them.

Using a Strength-Based Approach

Within the primary care setting, the clinician becomes familiar with a child's strengths and challenges. They can articulate and celebrate an autistic child's strengths along with the family and use these strengths to help identify mechanisms for encouraging the child. If a child is averse to reading, for example, suggesting books about topics of interest to the child may be helpful. A child struggling with fine motor skills or handwriting might be allowed to write about their favorite topic or be given access to their preferred interest after a challenging lesson. A child's strengths might be highlighted to the class in presentations or in specific jobs within the classroom to help the child with peer engagement. For example, the very active child might be given the job of getting up to turn off the lights, the child interested in putting things away might be the teacher's helper, and the child with a specific area of expertise might be paired with a classmate struggling in that area. Highlighting a child's strengths will promote motivation and self-esteem as well as support constructive peer engagement.

This type of strength-based approach can build on a child's skills to find social, academic, and, eventually, vocational opportunities. The hope is that the family, professionals caring for the child, and those in the child's environment will learn to cherish the earnestness, the caring, and the unique attributes that the child exhibits. The pediatric primary care clinician is able to support the developmental process and help peel away the barriers that children on the autism spectrum can face in finding their paths. Clinicians should focus on the view that children on the spectrum are not individuals who need to be fixed but individuals who benefit from adaptation of their environments to allow for new skill acquisition and enhanced experiences throughout the lifespan. The goal should be to find opportunities for meaningful and purposeful engagement in social, academic, and vocational pathways. The primary care clinician is uniquely situated to be able to observe and celebrate successes while supporting the process of prioritizing goals and therapies that strengthen the child and the family. Doing so supports the family's ability to find hope and resilience for the future as they build on their child's strengths. Pediatric primary care clinicians are not expected to be autism experts, but listening, observing, and using pediatric skills will positively affect the care that children on the spectrum receive. The case vignette presented at the start of this chapter represents an optimal model of care for a child on the spectrum in a practice that uses effective principles of chronic care management.

Clinical Pearls

In the child who receives a diagnosis of autism, it is likely that a complexity of developmental, behavioral, and medical health conditions will develop that require monitoring, accommodations, and intervention.

- There is no "one size fits all" approach to autism.
- Ongoing care requires an understanding of who the individual is, what the family needs, and what is known about autism.
- As a priority, the pediatric primary care clinician should create the opportunity for listening to and fostering partnerships with parents.
- Children on the autism spectrum frequently use health care services but are less likely than their neurotypical peers to receive vaccines and preventive care.
- The pediatric primary care clinician along with the other members of the child's team should coordinate the care the child receives.

References

Carbone PS, Murphy NA, Norlin C, Azor V, Sheng X, Young PC. Parent and pediatrician perspectives regarding the primary care of children with autism spectrum disorders. *J Autism Dev Disord.* 2013;43(4):964–972 PMID: 22948548 doi: 10.1007/s10803-012-1640-7

Cummings JR, Lynch FL, Rust KC, et al. Health services utilization among children with and without autism spectrum disorders. *J Autism Dev Disord.* 2016;46(3):910–920 PMID: 26547921 doi: 10.1007/s10803-015-2634-z

Da Paz NS, Siegel B, Coccia MA, Epel ES. Acceptance or despair? maternal adjustment to having a child diagnosed with autism. *J Autism Dev Disord.* 2018;48(6):1971–1981 PMID: 29307036 doi: 10.1007/s10803-017-3450-4

Foy JM, Green CM, Earls MF, et al; American Academy of Pediatrics Committee on Psychosocial Aspects of Child and Family Health and Mental Health Leadership Work Group. Mental health competencies for pediatric practice. *Pediatrics.* 2019;144(5):e20192757 PMID: 31636143 doi: 10.1542/peds.2019-2757

Maenner MJ, Warren Z, Williams AR, et al. Prevalence and characteristics of autism spectrum disorder among children aged 8 years—Autism and Developmental Disabilities Monitoring Network, 11 sites, United States, 2020. *MMWR Surveill Summ.* 2023;72(2):1–14 PMID: 36952288 doi: 10.15585/mmwr.ss7202a1

Mazurek MO, Harkins C, Menezes M, et al. Primary care providers' perceived barriers and needs for support in caring for children with autism. *J Pediatr.* 2020;221:240–245.e1 PMID: 32143927 doi: 10.1016/j.jpeds.2020.01.014

Mazurek MO, Parker RA, Chan J, Kuhlthau K, Sohl K; ECHO Autism Collaborative. Effectiveness of the Extension for Community Health Outcomes model as applied to primary care for autism: a partial stepped-wedge randomized clinical trial. *JAMA Pediatr.* 2020;174(5):e196306 PMID: 32150229 doi: 10.1001/jamapediatrics.2019.6306

Stahmer AC, Mandell DS. State infant/toddler program policies for eligibility and services provision for young children with autism. *Adm Policy Ment Health.* 2007;34(1):29–37 PMID: 16758329 doi: 10.1007/s10488-006-0060-4

CHAPTER

2

Demographics, Etiology, and Clinical Presentation

CASE VIGNETTE

A family visits a pediatric practice for the first time with their 2-year-old child for a health supervision visit. Both parents are 42 years old and have dedicated careers as computer programmers. They report that their child met all developmental milestones on surveillance and screening, but at today's visit, the parents' response on autism-specific screening raises concern for possible autism. When this response is explored, the parents share that their child is very intelligent and occupies himself with alphabet blocks while they work from home. They also share that he becomes absorbed in his play and does not typically respond when they call his name. The child can label all letters, numbers, colors, and shapes on multiple electronic games. The parents have an older child who is being treated for attention-deficit/hyperactivity disorder and excels academically. Although that child demonstrates strong academic abilities, his school has expressed some concern for his lack of social engagement and some externalizing behaviors exhibited during lunch and recess. There is a paternal uncle who was diagnosed with intellectual disability as a child, did not complete high school, and lives with his parents. The clinician considers the increased likelihood of autism in this child.

Autism typically manifests in early childhood, and its challenges may have significant and lifelong effects on the individual's ability to meet the demands of social, academic, and daily routines. Autism is defined by a group of behavioral manifestations delineated in the *Diagnostic and Statistical Manual of Mental Disorders, Fifth Edition, Text Revision* (*DSM-5-TR*), a reference that is revised periodically by a large group of experts who evaluate the reliability of the diagnostic criteria.

Autism is diagnosed across all geographic locations—within and outside the United States—ethnicities, races, and socioeconomic statuses. Reported prevalence rates have increased as diagnostic criteria change, awareness increases, and effective therapies become widely available. There is also evidence for diagnostic substitution of autism for intellectual disability (ID). Rates of primary ID have decreased from the 1990s to recent times. The Autism and Developmental Disabilities Monitoring (ADDM) Network tracks prevalence rates of autism among 4- and 8-year-olds within 11 communities of the United States by reviewing medical records. Although prevalence rates vary across the country, they are mostly stable across socioeconomic and racial groupings. Recent ADDM surveillance data indicate that autism prevalence among 8-year-olds is higher among children from several racial and ethnic groups, including Asian or Pacific Islander, American Indian or Alaska Native, non-Hispanic Black, Hispanic or Latino, and multiracial children. In addition, these prevalence rates are inversely related to the mean household income. Recently, the ADDM reported that all groups of children of color on the autism spectrum were more likely to be diagnosed with co-occurring ID and diagnosed later in life. This fact raises concern about potential bias or challenges with access to diagnostic services as well as added environmental risk factors that these children may experience. Discrepancies in diagnosis and access to care have been associated with the social drivers of care related to higher levels of poverty, including lack of transportation, housing instability, stressors to parental health and well-being, food insecurity, financial instability, lack of insurance, and poor experiences with the health care system.

The data from the Centers for Disease Control and Prevention demonstrated that between 2000 and 2023, the rate of autism increased from 1 in 149 to 1 in 31 among 8-year-old children. With these changes, there has been consistent male predominance, with a boy to girl ratio of 4:1. Increases in the number of children receiving a diagnosis of autism without associated ID have presumably resulted from the refinement of the diagnostic process as well as the broadening of diagnostic criteria.

The History of the Diagnosis

Autism was first described in the *DSM* in 1952 within the context of schizophrenia and then described as an independent entity in 1980. Autism was first referred to as "infantile autism," manifesting early in life, before 30 months of age. By 1987, the terminology was expanded to "autistic disorder," which was used to describe individuals with a "pervasive lack of responsiveness to people." It was not until the *DSM-IV* was published in 1994 that autistic disorder was divided into a wider variety of clinical entities with specific diagnostic criteria: autism, Asperger syndrome, pervasive developmental disorder not otherwise specified (PDD-NOS), and childhood disintegrative disorder. The children diagnosed with PDD-NOS did not meet criteria for a more specific diagnosis. Over time, it was observed that diagnoses of PDD-NOS and Asperger syndrome were not specific and were not stable over the lifespan. Individual diagnoses shifted between these subtypes, and individuals no longer met diagnostic criteria.

In 2013, the *DSM-5* redefined autism as a single broad entity of autism with or without co-occurring conditions such as intellectual and/or language disability (refer to Chapter 6, Establishing the Autism Diagnosis, for information on all aspects of diagnosing autism). A range of severity levels were described. These severity ratings are used to describe the amount of support needed for the child to be successful. Although their use is not recommended for young children as discussed in Chapter 6, when there is a need to describe the child's functioning, a careful description of their strengths and needs is helpful. The *DSM-5* diagnostic criteria are more specific and more stable than previous iterations, and although the subtypes are no longer used, individuals previously diagnosed with PDD-NOS or Asperger syndrome are still recognized as meeting criteria for an autism diagnosis.

Autism diagnoses will be made by professionals such as experienced neurologists, developmental pediatricians, general pediatricians, psychologists, or psychiatrists. There are no specifications on how an autism diagnosis is made and which specific tools must be used, but careful documentation of how the child meets *DSM* diagnostic criteria through the use of standardized diagnostic tools, structured observation of the child, and a thorough caregiver history is required and likely mandated by the insurance provider. Some diagnoses are made by interdisciplinary teams with reliance on the assessments of educators, speech pathologists, and other early childhood specialists. In settings where access to interdisciplinary teams is not available, the clinician will be called upon to obtain feedback from educators, caregivers, and allied health professionals familiar with the child, in addition to conducting their clinical assessment. The parameters of diagnosis should include an assessment of developmental/cognitive status, a physical examination, and an assessment for genetic and medical etiologies. An autism-specific tool should be administered to support the diagnosis. Some centers use what is considered the "gold standard": the Autism Diagnostic Observation Schedule, Second Edition (ADOS-2), with or without the Autism Diagnostic Interview, Revised (ADI-R). Others may use clinical expertise and rely on a variety of standardized checklists and questionnaires or a level II screener such as the Screening Tool for Autism in Toddlers and Young Children (STAT).

Etiology and Genetics

When approached as a clinical entity, autism represents a complex interaction between genetic phenomena or inheritance and the influence of environmental features or epigenetic mechanisms. It is clear there are genetic links or familial tendencies toward autism. The data guide the primary care clinician to have a raised index of suspicion when there is a family history of autism or a related disorder. Twin studies have shown a concordance rate of 98% in monozygotic twins and 53% to 67% in dizygotic twins. The likelihood in siblings in families with a child on the autism spectrum varies depending on the sex of the index child and the number of affected family members. The sibling's overall likelihood is roughly 20% if only one child is affected and 37% if multiple siblings are already affected. Females on the spectrum seem to carry a larger genetic load for a family. If the affected child is a girl, the likelihood of subsequent children receiving an autism diagnosis is higher.

Family members will often have traits, characteristics, or subthreshold characteristics of autism without meeting criteria for a full diagnosis. These traits can include cognitive challenges; tic disorder; anxiety; social, communication, or pragmatic language difficulties; executive function challenges; and attention-deficit/hyperactivity disorder.

Just as there is variability in the phenotypic expression of autism, there is a myriad of genetic variants and copy number variants (deletions or duplications of DNA regions) associated with autism. More than 800 genes and many genetic syndromes are associated with autism. Some individuals with the clinical diagnosis will have chromosomal deletions or duplications; some, identified genetic syndromes; and others, a single gene disorder that has been associated with autism. The finding of genetic alterations provides an opportunity for better understanding the likelihood of autism in the individual as well as provides the possibility of discovering new therapies in the future.

The yield on genetic testing remains low in the general population of individuals on the spectrum. When chromosomal microarray analysis (CMA) and whole exome sequencing are combined, as many as 15% of those on the spectrum will be found to have associated pathology, whereas CMA alone has a yield of 4% to 9%. Most variants are de novo except in cases where multiple family members are affected. The addition of minor physical malformations, or dysmorphisms, increases the yield of combined CMA and whole exome sequencing to 35%.

In 2011, the American College of Medical Genetics and Genomics recommended CMA and fragile X syndrome testing as a first-tier assessment for all children who receive an autism diagnosis. Despite this recommendation, the high cost of and inconsistency in insurance coverage limit the ability to make this recommendation a standard of care. Despite this limitation, finding a genetic link can be very helpful to the child and family. The link may better inform the prognosis of medical complexities associated with autism and, in some cases, offer a path for screening and treatment (eg, for cardiac or renal involvement). Further, the knowledge of a biological link can be helpful in providing the child a cohort of others with similar genetic makeup. The process of finding a cohort can result in many positive outcomes: receiving emotional and practical support from others affected, opportunities for research, and access to therapies specific to the genetic alterations.

The Influence of Epigenetics

Advanced parental age, high-risk perinatal factors, and environmental exposures are epigenetic factors that have clear additive effects on the likelihood of having a child on the autism spectrum. Recent studies have demonstrated an increased likelihood of autism after prenatal exposure to increased particulate matter, organophosphate pesticides, and maternal metabolic conditions such as diabetes. The mechanism by which these epigenetic factors contribute to a clinical condition such as autism is still investigative, but the exposure likely influences gene expression or neuronal development during the prenatal period.

There is evidence of structural brain differences in individuals on the spectrum. Some studies show abnormal overgrowth and organization of neurons, abnormal neural connectivity, decreased synapse density, or patchy areas of abnormal cerebral cortical architecture. Some of these structural differences likely occur early in pregnancy, and others could evolve over the individual's lived experiences. They tend to occur in the frontal and temporal lobes known to be involved in emotional regulation, social behavior, and language. This evidence supports the existence of biological differences in the brains of those on the spectrum, potentially identifying biomarkers that could enhance screening and diagnostic procedures. While these findings hold promise for future therapeutic applications, their current clinical utility remains limited, indicating a need for further research to translate these insights into effective supports and services for individuals on the spectrum.

Clinical Presentation of Autism

The clinical features of autism typically manifest early in life. The developmental trajectory of a child who later receives an autism diagnosis follows that of a typically developing child until around 14 months of age, at which time expressive language and affect sharing will begin to deviate. Features indicating a need for referral early in infancy (increased head lag, clumsiness, decreased or misdirected eye contact, lack of babbling, or low core tone) have been identified but are not accurate predictors of later autism.

Developmental screening tools typically used in primary care settings are not sensitive enough to detect subtly atypical social-emotional development in an autistic child's infancy. It is not until the second year after birth that these tools become likely to identify nonspecific developmental deviations as they become more pronounced. For this reason, the American Academy of Pediatrics has recommended autism-specific screening at the 18- and 24-month health supervision visits. This is addressed in Chapter 5, Autism Screening in Primary Care.

The earliest findings suggestive of autism are those resulting from delays in communication and joint attention along with the presence of restricted and repetitive behaviors. These early features of autism are summarized in **Box 2.1**. Chapter 3, Joint Attention: What Is It and Why Is It Important?, discusses joint attention in detail.

BOX 2.1 Early Features of Autism in the 18- to 24-Month-Old Child

Communication

- Not responding to name by 12 months
- Little response to verbal instructions
- Not pointing or using gesture
- Lack of vocal sounds to make requests
- Restricted or regressed vocalizations
- Echolalia

Social Behavior

- Decreased or misdirected eye contact
- Not sharing things or interests
- Lack of engagement with others
- Absent shared smile
- Limited imitation
- Use of a person's hand to obtain what they want

Stereotypical Behavior

- Repetitive behavior, rituals, or atypical interests
- Unusual attachments to or use of objects, routines, or toys
- Repetitive lining up or arranging of objects
- Atypical sensory responses
- Stereotypical movements such as toe walking or hand flapping
- Lack of play skills

Other Behavior

- Lack of play themes
- Low core tone; head lag
- Motor coordination challenges
- Developmental regression

Children may reliably receive a diagnosis of autism as early as 18 months of age, although many will not meet criteria for a diagnosis until later. Of those who received a diagnosis at age 36 months, 63% of diagnoses were missed at age 18 months and 41% were missed at age 24 months. The stability of the diagnosis is less in those who received a diagnosis before 3 years of age: 82.6% of children who received it at 18 months met criteria for persistent diagnosis at 3 years, while 91.8% of children who received it at 2 years had persistent features. Despite these data, many autism specialists will be comfortable diagnosing autism in a child during the second year after birth if they meet all diagnostic criteria, realizing that many will not meet criteria for a full diagnosis until after their third birthday. Children who continue to have atypical but subthreshold features of autism require ongoing monitoring for the development of autism and other developmental conditions.

The older preschooler who has not yet received a diagnosis of autism may present with a variety of behavioral features (**Box 2.2**). Without suspicion for autism, a child with this type of presentation may be treated only for behavior that is disruptive to one's functioning or others' space, without an understanding of the etiology of the behavior.

BOX 2.2 Features of Autism in Older Preschoolers

- Difficulty with transitions
- Aggression
- Emotional dysregulation
- Difficulty sharing
- Difficulty engaging peers
- More time spent in solitary exploration
- Difficulty staying seated
- Not engaging in activities
- Eloping
- Not asking for help or making requests
- Divergence from developmental milestones that suggests the need for supportive strategies
- Behavior that others find disruptive
- Struggling to follow instruction
- Picky eating
- Poor sleep

Late Diagnoses

Despite the attention to careful surveillance and screening for autism, some individuals on the spectrum will not receive a diagnosis until later childhood or even adulthood, when the demands of the environment exceed their developmental abilities. The lack of identification and access to therapeutic support may put these individuals at greater risk for secondary behavioral health sequelae. There is well-documented evidence that females tend to receive autism diagnoses later than their male counterparts. Females are less likely to be identified by teachers and other professionals and may present for assessment later, when the challenges require more support. In general, girls seem to have a more specific female phenotype that involves a higher degree of social engagement, improved peer relations, and fewer repetitive and externalizing behaviors but more internalizing behaviors. The internalizing behaviors create a vulnerability for these females for anxiety, depression, and eating disorders, and families may seek evaluation for these issues first.

Individuals receiving a diagnosis later in life tend to have stronger language or cognitive abilities and more academic strengths. They are likely to require a comprehensive psychological evaluation addressing a complexity of differential diagnoses to better understand the cause of the presenting concerns.

Autism tends to affect the health and well-being of the child and their entire family. Many behaviors indicative of autism develop very early in a child's life, while other autistic features will not become apparent until later in life. It is incumbent on the pediatric primary care clinician to remain ever vigilant as concerns are shared and characteristics evolve. The chapter case vignette highlights the necessity of integrating family-reported concerns and risk factors with ongoing developmental surveillance, autism-specific screening, and knowledge of the developmental course of autism to inform comprehensive care for children and their families.

Clinical Pearls

- Autism is common and occurs across all ethnicities, races, and socioeconomic groups.
- Of 8-year-old children, 1 in 31 receives a diagnosis of autism.
- Boys receive a diagnosis of autism more commonly than girls, with a ratio of 4:1.
- There is a strong genetic link in autism: In families with one child who has received a diagnosis, 20% of siblings will be affected. When multiple children in a family have received a diagnosis, 37% of siblings will likely show features of autism.
- The combination of CMA and whole exome sequencing may be used to demonstrate associated genetic links.
- A diagnosis of autism is reliable as early as 18 months of age but more stable after 24 to 30 months of age.
- Children who have an increased likelihood of autism but who do not meet diagnostic criteria should be monitored for later diagnosis or developmental challenges requiring support.

References

Bargiela S, Steward R, Mandy W. The experiences of late-diagnosed women with autism spectrum conditions: an investigation of the female autism phenotype. *J Autism Dev Disord.* 2016;46(10):3281–3294 PMID: 27457364 doi: 10.1007/s10803-016-2872-8

Bourson L, Prevost C. Characteristics of restricted interests in girls with ASD compared to boys: a systematic review of the literature. *Eur Child Adolesc Psychiatry.* 2024;33(4):987–1004 PMID: 35644857 doi: 10.1007/s00787-022-01998-5

Brian JA, Zwaigenbaum L, Ip A. Standards of diagnostic assessment for autism spectrum disorder. *Paediatr Child Health.* 2019;24(7):444–451 PMID: 31660042 doi: 10.1093/pch/pxz117

Carbone PS, Campbell K, Wilkes J, et al. Primary care autism screening and later autism diagnosis. *Pediatrics.* 2020;146(2):e20192314 PMID: 32632024 doi: 10.1542/peds.2019-2314

Centers for Disease Control and Prevention. Autism and Developmental Disabilities Monitoring (ADDM) Network. Autism Spectrum Disorder (ASD). May 27, 2025. Accessed February 26, 2026. https://www.cdc.gov/autism/addm-network

Chiarotti F, Venerosi A. Epidemiology of autism spectrum disorders: a review of worldwide prevalence estimates since 2014. *Brain Sci.* 2020;10(5):274 PMID: 32370097 doi: 10.3390/brainsci10050274

Constantino JN, Abbacchi AM, Saulnier C, et al. Timing of the diagnosis of autism in African American children. *Pediatrics.* 2020;146(3):e20193629 PMID: 32839243 doi: 10.1542/peds.2019-3629

Di Renzo M, Guerriero V, Zavattini GC, Petrillo M, Racinaro L, Bianchi di Castelbianco F. Parental attunement, insightfulness, and acceptance of child diagnosis in parents of children with autism: clinical implications. *Front Psychol.* 2020;11:1849 PMID: 32849089 doi: 10.3389/fpsyg.2020.01849

Gabrielsen TP, Farley M, Speer L, Villalobos M, Baker CN, Miller J. Identifying autism in a brief observation. *Pediatrics.* 2015;135(2):e330–e338 PMID: 25583913 doi: 10.1542/peds.2014-1428

Genovese A, Butler MG. The autism spectrum: behavioral, psychiatric and genetic associations. *Genes (Basel).* 2023;14(3):677 PMID: 36980949 doi: 10.3390/genes14030677

Guan X, Zwaigenbaum L, Sonnenberg LK. Building capacity for community pediatric autism diagnosis: a systemic review of physician training programs. *J Dev Behav Pediatr.* 2022;43(1):44–54 PMID: 34907998 doi: 10.1097/DBP.0000000000001042

Harstad E, Hanson E, Brewster SJ, et al. Persistence of autism spectrum disorder from early childhood through school age. *JAMA Pediatr.* 2023;177(11):1197–1205 PMID: 37782510 doi: 10.1001/jamapediatrics.2023.4003

Hyman SL, Levy SE, Myers SM, et al; American Academy of Pediatrics Council on Children With Disabilities and Section on Developmental and Behavioral Pediatrics. Identification, evaluation, and management of children with autism spectrum disorder. *Pediatrics.* 2020;145(1):e20193447 PMID: 31843864 doi: 10.1542/peds.2019-3447

Jin T, Pang Q, Huang W, et al. Particulate matter 2.5 causally increased genetic risk of autism spectrum disorder. *BMC Psychiatry.* 2024;24(1):129 PMID: 38365642 doi: 10.1186/s12888-024-05564-y

Landa RJ. Diagnosis of autism spectrum disorders in the first 3 years of life. *Nat Clin Pract Neurol.* 2008;4(3):138–147 PMID: 18253102 doi: 10.1038/ncpneuro0731

Ozonoff S, Young GS, Bradshaw J, et al. Familial recurrence of autism: updates from the Baby Siblings Research Consortium. *Pediatrics.* 2024;154(2):e2023065297 PMID: 39011552 doi: 10.1542/peds.2023-065297

Román P, Ruiz-González C, Rueda-Ruzafa L, Cardona D, Requena M, Alarcón R. Exposure to environmental pesticides and the risk of autism spectrum disorders: a population-based case-control study. *Medicina (Kaunas).* 2024;60(3):479 PMID: 38541205 doi: 10.3390/medicina60030479

Zwaigenbaum L, Bauman ML, Stone WL, et al. Early identification of autism spectrum disorder: recommendations for practice and research. *Pediatrics.* 2015;136(suppl 1):S10–S40 PMID: 26430168 doi: 10.1542/peds.2014-3667C

Zwaigenbaum L, Bryson SE, Brian J, et al. Stability of diagnostic assessment for autism spectrum disorder between 18 and 36 months in a high-risk cohort. *Autism Res.* 2016;9(7):790–800 PMID: 26613202 doi: 10.1002/aur.1585

CHAPTER

3

Joint Attention: What Is It and Why Is It Important?

CASE VIGNETTE

At a 2-year health supervision visit, a parent raises concern that their child might be autistic. The parent reports that their child speaks no words, and they are anxious to get their child help. Autism screening performed in the office using the Modified Checklist for Autism in Toddlers, Revised with Follow-Up (M-CHAT-R/F) does not identify any significant concern, and the history reveals no atypical restricted or repetitive behavioral features or family history of autism or related disorders. The pediatric primary care clinician learns that the child seems to understand verbal commands and responds to being called. The child makes some babbling sounds, and a few of them seem to have intent for communication and accompany the use of gesture, but he does not speak any words. The clinician uses the remainder of the visit to assess the child's skills of social engagement and joint attention to address the parent's concern for possible autism.

What Is Joint Attention?

Joint attention describes a series of preverbal behaviors that evolve from as early as 6 months of age and are firmly established by 18 months of age. These skills provide the foundation for successful communication and social engagement. Joint attention occurs when 2 individuals share interest in a common object or event and are aware of this sharing. These skills are developed by a child as they learn to combine the use of gesture with pointing, eye contact, and gaze shifting from an object to a communication partner. Eventually, the child will add the use of vocalizations, and, later, specific words, to facilitate the interaction. Early delays in joint attention put children at risk for communication challenges and can be the first indicator of an evolving picture of autism. Support targeting joint attention leads to improved communication. It is important for pediatric clinicians to become familiar with this developmental process to identify children with an increased likelihood of autism and other conditions that may lead to social communication delays and refer them for support when concern is raised. It should be noted that cultural differences can significantly influence eye contact behaviors. In some cultures, direct eye gaze may be considered attentive and respectful, while in others, it may be seen as intrusive or disrespectful. As a result, mutual eye gaze may appear differently in some cultures than what is usually seen in many Western cultures.

Why Is Joint Attention Important?

Joint attention skills are strongly associated with successful social communication and engagement and signify that the young child has learned they can effectively get their needs met by interacting with another individual. These skills are necessary for early learning and social interaction. The first evidence of intentional communication in a typically developing child occurs at 9 months of age. The child shifts eye gaze from the adult to the desired object and is able to follow the adult's gaze to share an experience of visual regard. A more mature requesting behavior can be observed when the child uses a vocalization or specific gesture until the desired outcome is obtained. The child's vocalizations evolve from nonspecific utterances to sounds that are more specific to the outcome (first a shriek and later a word approximation). The child's nonverbal behaviors, a reach or, later, a point, signify specific intent and are intact by 12 months of age. Between 13 and 15 months of age, the child combines pointing with gaze shifting to make requests for things (protoimperative pointing), and by 18 months of age, toddlers can be seen in joint attention with their caregiver up to 26% of playtime. By this developmental level, pointing is used not only to make requests but to share interest and comments (protodeclarative pointing). **Box 3.1** outlines the stages of joint attention.

BOX 3.1 The Stages of Joint Attention

1. Infant shares eye contact with others and engages in back-and-forth games.
2. Infant follows the adult's gaze when an object is within sight and, later, when it is not within sight.
3. Infant initiates directing the attention of others through gaze shifting (ie, looking at the object, looking back to the parent).
4. Infant learns to coordinate the use of gesture first, followed by the use of words, to direct and share attention.
5. Infant uses joint attention to make requests and, later, to share and obtain feedback from others.

Joint Attention: Key Features in Autism

As a child matures, joint attention is used repeatedly to initiate and maintain social interaction and share interests. It is through this type of social engagement and play that a child learns to share, take turns, and effectively problem-solve. Children on the autism spectrum are less likely to engage socially and may therefore miss out on the learning that occurs through interpersonal relationships. The lack of these joint attention skills is an early feature indicating a need for referral that might be present in the young child who receives a diagnosis of autism.

The absence of joint attention may manifest by a lack of showing, bringing, initiating interaction around, responding to, or pointing out objects of desire. Parents may report that their child on the spectrum does not use gestures and does not follow a point. Children on the spectrum tend to be independent, to play alone, and to initiate interaction infrequently and may lack the skills of social reciprocity that occur through play. They tend not to show what they enjoy or want to share with others. Children on the spectrum may pull the body of a parent toward the object of desire, using the parent's body to obtain what they want rather than using a form of communication to engage the parent and make their needs known.

Children on the spectrum may learn rote language skills and have strengths in reciting lines or labels from books, videos, or songs. They might have a large vocabulary they use to label objects around them. They might learn to identify colors, to recite the alphabet, or to read while not yet having the ability to process or understand what they are reading. These skills are often not used in conjunction with sharing with a partner in a back-and-forth fashion and can be part of a child's specific or focused interests. In this type of language use, the child is unable to take turns in conversation and instead may be focused on talking about what they are interested in. They might use language they have heard others use or echo phrases from videos, songs, or poems. They might struggle to answer "wh" (what, where, why, when, and who) questions or build on conversation that others initiate. Often there is a very narrow repertoire of conversational exchange focused on functional need or specific interests. For example, a child with a keen interest in opening and closing doors might be observed making eye contact and asking to "open doors" but might show limited variety in communicative efforts.

The lack of early joint attention skills is a sensitive but nonspecific predictor of autism. Delays in joint attention skills are associated with many types of communication, social, adaptive, and cognitive delays seen in elementary school–aged children and therefore indicate a need for support and monitoring. Other developmental conditions, being deaf or hard of hearing, social-emotional trauma, or social anxiety need to be distinguished from this evolving picture of autism. Children who are hard of hearing may appear to have diminished responsiveness and joint attention, especially if their parents are deaf or hard of hearing. They are likely to demonstrate a visual vigilance that they use to attempt to compensate for their lack of auditory cues. Children with social anxiety will demonstrate strengths in familiar environments but not in new settings. Other children, who are later diagnosed with intellectual disabilities, are likely to have more developmental delays in addition to those of joint attention.

Support for Delays in Joint Attention

Primary care clinicians should inquire more specifically about a child's communicative use of language and distinguish whether or not the child uses language associated with social interaction. It is important for a pediatric primary care clinician to inquire about and observe the child in a variety of situations and structured types of interaction to better understand the child's joint attention abilities and possible need for support. This is discussed in more detail in Chapter 6, Establishing the Autism Diagnosis. If concern is identified, providing guidelines on promoting play and skills of social engagement can be beneficial. Often the act of removing screens and toys with computerized operations and spending more time in face-to-face playtime with a child can significantly strengthen development (refer to the section How can I support my child? in Appendix B, Parent Handout: What Is Autism and How Do I Know if My Preschool-Aged Child Is on the Spectrum?).

Pediatric primary care clinicians can provide support for parents in distinguishing between rote language skills and those used for meaningful, functional communication. This can be accomplished through direct observation in the office or with targeted questions about the child's language use in daily life. For example, does the child use language to share interests, make requests, or ask for help? Is the language focused on repeating sequences of numbers or naming objects of interest?

Clinicians can offer valuable guidance on the importance of joint attention, reciprocal conversation, and play in early communication development. Recommending specific types of toys and interactive play strategies can help parents foster joint attention skills (refer to the section How can I support my child? in Appendix B, Parent Handout: What Is Autism and How Do I Know if My Preschool-Aged Child Is on the Spectrum?). This guidance is crucial in helping parents recognize that an emphasis on rote memorization or screen-based learning is insufficient for children with early social and communication delays. Instead, these children benefit most from interactive and relationship-based learning experiences that support their communication development.

Many support programs for young children on the autism spectrum include components targeting joint attention. These are best taught by speech pathologists and early intervention specialists, although many applied behavior analysis programs include these goals as well. Early intervention specialists have expertise in play, social engagement, and joint attention, so a referral for services is a logical first step when there is identified risk for delays in these areas. Pediatric primary care clinicians working with young children with such delays should learn to identify private specialists in their area who specialize in working on social engagement and joint attention. In addition, there are many resources that can be shared with parents to help guide how they can structure play and interaction with their child to support the development of these skills.

Specific approaches to teaching joint attention in children on the spectrum and resources for parents are listed in **Box 3.2** and discussed in more detail in Chapter 8, Evidence-Based Supports and Services. Efficacy has been demonstrated by multiple supports and services, such as the Early Start Denver Model, as well as by many peer model supports and services. It should be noted that the availability of specialists in these areas varies across the country.

BOX 3.2 Parent Resources for Developing Joint Attention Skills

- Language and literacy tips from The Hanen Centre: www.hanen.org/information-tips?Handouts=true
- Promoting parent-mediated child learning opportunities; 4 learning modules for parents from Help is in Your Hands: www.helpisinyourhands.org (free registration)
- Handouts for parents provided in Appendix B, Parent Handout: What Is Autism and How Do I Know if My Preschool-Aged Child Is on the Spectrum? and Appendix F, Parent Resources on Autism
- Referral for speech therapy or early intervention services

Strategies clinicians can share with parents can be summarized as follows:

- Encourage face-to-face interaction.
- Remove distractions, including anything with batteries or electronics.
- Put your child's preferred toys out of reach so they need to "ask" for help to obtain them.
- Find toys and play that capture your child's attention.
- Provide extra time between each interaction to allow your child an opportunity to use their skills.
- Observe which sensory stimuli promote attention and which cause aversion in your child.
- Imitate your child's actions.
- Respond to your child's attempts to communicate.
- Use simple 1- to 2-word phrases to teach and avoid overwhelming your child.
- Play games involving physical interaction that are appealing to your child.
- Model what you want the response to be.
- Make book reading fun and interactive.

For more information, refer to Appendix B, Parent Handout: What Is Autism and How Do I Know if My Preschool-Aged Child Is on the Spectrum?

There are evidence-based curricula focused on teaching social engagement and communication that are available to professionals and parents. The Early Start Denver Model is an example of one such curriculum. Teaching modules and courses for parents and professionals are available through select providers and on the internet (www.esdm.co). Many other curricula are used widely and provide practical and helpful tools that do not yet have the rigor of data to support their efficacy. Examples include The Hanen Centre (including the language and literacy tips from its website and methods from *More Than Words* by Fern Sussman), DIRFloortime (from the Developmental, Individual-differences, and Relationship-based model), and SCERTS (Social Communication, Emotional Regulation, and Transactional Support). If a child receives an autism diagnosis, a more comprehensive care plan should be put into place targeting a broader array of developmental domains. This is addressed in Chapter 8, Evidence-Based Supports and Services.

The case vignette presented at the start of this chapter provides an example of how the pediatric primary care clinician is able to focus the assessment of a child on joint attention, social engagement, and communication as possible early indicators of autism even before the child meets diagnostic criteria. This is the ideal approach to determining the likelihood of autism as well as a possible need for referral for diagnostic testing and support.

CASE VIGNETTE: CONCLUSION

The primary care clinician observes the parent interacting with the child and notices the following behaviors: the child responds to their name being called and to simple verbal requests, the child makes eye contact with a shared smile with both parent and clinician, the child points and grunts to show interest in something or to make a request, the child follows the parent's point and retrieves an object to bring it to the parent for play, the child enjoys sitting in back-and-forth play and uses objects in typical types of play (ie, rolling a car, rocking and feeding a baby, pretending to talk on the phone with a block), and, on request, the child will imitate actions modeled by the clinician ("Now you do this!"). The clinician reassures the parent that the child has many healthy developmental skills, but he has an expressive language delay. Although there is no specific concern for autism, the clinician refers the child for speech therapy. A variety of handouts and links are provided to the parent to help guide their interactions and play with their child in the interim. The clinician will have the child return regularly to monitor his developmental progress and response to therapy to determine if a more comprehensive assessment or support is indicated.

Clinical Pearls

Joint attention is

- The ability to follow, join, and initiate attention and interaction
- Necessary to share attention with another human
- Used to share intent and affect to allow engagement
- Used by a child to get their needs met
- Necessary for cognitive and social learning
- A foundation for teaching and learning
- Correlated with language acquisition and the ability to understand that others have intentions

Delays in joint attention may be the first indicator of autism and provide an opportunity for support before a diagnosis is made. The pediatric primary care clinician can provide the parent with helpful tips on promoting joint attention through play while waiting for a referral to an early childhood specialist.

References

Bruinsma Y, Koegel RL, Koegel LK. Joint attention and children with autism: a review of the literature. *Ment Retard Dev Disabil Res Rev.* 2004;10(3):169–175 PMID: 15611988 doi: 10.1002/mrdd.20036

Franchini M, Armstrong VL, Schaer M, Smith IM. Initiation of joint attention and related visual attention processes in infants with autism spectrum disorder: literature review. *Child Neuropsychol.* 2019;25(3):287–317 PMID: 30041581 doi: 10.1080/09297049.2018.1490706

Kourassanis-Velasquez J, Jones EA. Increasing joint attention in children with autism and their peers. *Behav Anal Pract.* 2018;12(1):78–94 PMID: 30918772 doi: 10.1007/s40617-018-0228-x

Sano M, Yoshimura Y, Hirosawa T, et al. Joint attention and intelligence in children with autism spectrum disorder without severe intellectual disability. *Autism Res.* 2021;14(12):2603–2612 PMID: 34427050 doi: 10.1002/aur.2600

CHAPTER 4

The Pragmatics of the Pediatric Visit

CASE VIGNETTE

It is late afternoon and the pediatrician is behind schedule. The nurse communicates that the next scheduled patient has been running in the hall and loudly singing the theme song from a popular children's movie. The nurse is unable to engage him, obtain vital signs, or successfully encourage him to enter the examination room. The parent is working hard to comfort the child, who is anxious, and some people in the waiting area seem uncomfortable.

Children on the autism spectrum and with other neurodevelopmental conditions are more likely to experience stress during a pediatric visit. This can lead to frustration for the professionals, the child, and the parent. The child's difficulty in meeting visit expectations may hinder both the exchange of information and the achievement of the visit's goals. When protocols are adapted for children on the spectrum and accommodations in the environment are put into place, a more successful experience can be had by all involved, who are now able to focus on the details of the health supervision visit.

Medical visits can be distressing to many children on the spectrum because these visits present unfamiliar expectations, changes in routine, a high sensory load, and new procedures that can be frightening to children. For children who prefer predictability and familiarity, these visits can produce anxiety. These children may already have anxiety caused by difficult experiences they have had in the medical system. If autistic children are feeling dysregulated in the medical setting, they may use coping behaviors such as making repetitive sounds or motor behaviors and may express their distress in atypical manners that others may mistakenly interpret as disruptive, such as running, climbing, making loud vocalizations, or seeking calming experiences.

Weitzman and colleagues describe the Supporting Access for Everyone Initiative that established principles of health care to address the challenges children with neurodevelopmental disabilities (NDDs) experience when their families are seeking health care. Their recommendations are based on the belief that all people deserve health care that is "accessible, human, and effective." This consensus statement outlines the aspects of care that contribute to the disparities experienced by children with NDDs, including practices that undervalue people with disabilities, a lack of training for health care professionals, and inequitable systems of care.

To create a more equitable health care system, the unique needs of each child and family must be thoughtfully integrated into every pediatric visit. Accommodations made to the environment and protocols involved in the pediatric visit can result in a significantly different experience for the child with a disability or neurodivergence. This will involve the use of a system of individualized and proactive planning, scheduling, and preparation. A care team at the practice will address these protocols over several visits. Feedback from the child and family is a necessary component of planning. All staff will benefit from training to ensure their understanding and approach to the autistic child is in sync with the philosophy of the practice. It is important that each clinician learn to value the experience of the autistic child and approach their care by assessing the need to support, accept, and include them in the visit. This philosophy of care results in a more respectful and inclusive experience.

Clinicians may discover that preparation for visits requires additional time and involvement of a team approach that extends beyond the actual visit. This can be costly, and finding ways to bill for extra time will encourage the practice to support children on the spectrum and their families.

Scheduling the Visit

It can be extremely effective to have protocols in the practice for scheduling visits for the child with a disability or neurodivergence. Assigning front desk and administrative staff to ask routine questions about relevant issues and establishing a process for documenting the responses in a designated, secure, and visible place in the child's health record can make each subsequent visit more comfortable for the child. In larger practices, it may be more appropriate to have nurses and clinicians collectively observe and collect information about a child's sensitivities, anxieties, and calming strategies at visits and designate which type of scheduling specifics need to be taken into account by the scheduler, as discussed in the following sections.

Questions Staff Can Be Trained to Routinely Ask Parents When Scheduling a Health Supervision Visit

Clinicians can begin by training appropriate staff to routinely ask the following questions when scheduling children for a health supervision visit:

- Does your child have developmental or behavioral needs that would benefit from consideration before the visit? Does your child tend to struggle during health supervision visits?
- Does your child have specific sensitivities, communication challenges, or fears that may make a pediatric visit more difficult? Are there specific triggers for your child's stress (sound, touch, space, certain types of experiences, or visuals)? How do you suggest managing each step? What strategies are helpful for comforting your child?

All staff and clinicians should have access to and be able to modify the notes about the child's specific needs at any contact point.

Scheduling Considerations

The following considerations can be helpful when scheduling a visit for a child with developmental challenges:

- Consider scheduling health supervision visits at the beginning of the morning or afternoon to minimize waiting and give extra time for each visit. Ask the parent what will be optimal for their child.
- Avoid scheduling a health supervision visit during a child's nap time.
- Prioritize continuity with clinicians and staff (if possible) to foster relationship building, trust, and familiarity.
- Consider whether the child would benefit from a brief nurse-only visit to become familiar with the office, the steps of the visit, and the staff before the health supervision appointment.
- Allow the family to prioritize telehealth visits when possible.

Preparing for Office Visits

The following preparation strategies can help support successful office visits and optimal care for children on the autism spectrum and their families:

- **Schedule visits for the autistic child at least every 6 months.** Clinicians may decide to schedule visits for the autistic child at a minimum of 6-month intervals to allow for time to focus only on issues related to autism or may consider a telehealth visit for the second annual visit to allow the child to be in a familiar and comfortable environment.

- **Use a care navigator.** The availability of staff operating as patient navigators can further support the child and family as they navigate a pediatric visit and community resources. Although care navigators may not always be readily available, this approach is a low-cost way to effectively support families. These individuals may be health care professionals who bill for their time or may be salaried paraprofessionals who have expertise in community resources and the needs of the family. They may be available through nonprofit organizations supporting individuals with disabilities or neurodivergence, parent support resources, academic specialty programs, or larger practices. For example, in the state of Virginia, funding supports free access to pediatric care navigators through the Virginia Mental Health Access Program. Care navigators can serve to understand the needs of families with children on the spectrum and then become familiar with and develop relationships with the schools, therapy centers, advocacy groups, and private therapies in the community. Care navigators can be an invaluable resource to parents by assisting families as they navigate insurance claims processes. Clinicians should ensure that the care navigator requests that parents bring reports and progress notes from all specialists and allied health professionals to health supervision visits for review. Care navigators should be included in team care management planning by managing referrals, questions, and follow-up after each visit for children on the spectrum.
- **Ensure that clinicians and staff are familiar with local autism resources, and compile lists of these resources to share with families.** These resources should include online national resources specific to autism, local autism specialists, autism-trained professionals, and early intervention resources. The list should specify whether these programs are publicly funded and available or have insurance restrictions. In addition, including advocacy resources available for families as they navigate services and the special education processes is helpful. There are likely to be a variety of parent-led autism resources in the community as well as nonprofit organizations that can assist with care navigation. A list of resources may be found in Appendix F, Parent Resources on Autism.
- **Implement strategies for documentation.** Clinicians should develop strategies for keeping track of relevant documents (eg, individualized education programs [IEPs], care plans, assessments) and monitoring the child's progress in the health record. Refer to Appendix A, Autism Monitoring Tool for the Pediatric Primary Care Clinician. This tool can be adapted for use in electronic health records (EHRs) or as a saved document ready for use at each visit. Many chapters in this book have tools for screening and documentation that can also be used when evaluating specific areas of challenge or that can be printed to share with the family.
- **Have the parent bring special education documents to each visit.** These documents should include psychological and educational testing results

obtained by the school system or in a private setting, the annual full IEP, and the IEP progress reports that parents receive quarterly. These documents should be entered into the health record so the clinician can review them with the family. The pediatric primary care clinician should become familiar with using these documents to understand the child's progress, their educational goals, and the methods being used (refer to Chapter 14, Working With Special Education Services: A Primer).

- **Craft a family-specific communication plan.** Allow the family/patient to choose their preferred mode of communication when not in person (telephone call, text, or voicemail) and when in person (to include augmentative forms of communication).

The Autism Friendly Initiative at Boston Medical Center offers more ideas for individualizing care in the medical setting (www.bmc.org/visiting-us/autism-friendly-initiative).

Guiding Families to Prepare for the Visit

Pediatric primary care clinicians can support families in preparing their child for the pediatric visit. There are strategies that support success for all young children coming to see their clinician, and families are likely to have ideas that should be considered. These strategies can be reviewed at each visit, and additional recommendations may be made when needed. To help children on the autism spectrum prepare for office visits, clinicians can suggest that families consider the following approaches:

- **Read books about going to the doctor.** Parents may choose to purchase a book, find a resource online, or make their own tool specific to their child's particular experiences and responses. These stories should provide a social story or script for a child so they understand what will happen at the visit. Resources to aid parents as they prepare their child for a visit to the doctor can be found on the Children's Hospital of Philadelphia website (www.chop.edu/centers-programs/child-life-education-and-creative-arts-therapy/prepare-your-child-visit-doctor) and the Autism Speaks website (www.autismspeaks.org/expert-opinion/autism-and-doctor-visits-family-seeks-help-ease-daughters-fears).
- **Show the child pictures of the clinicians, staff, and office space.** Clinicians can consider posting pictures on the practice's website for parents to access.
- **Make a visual schedule of the doctor visit.** A visual schedule breaks the visit into a series of actions and represents them in a visual manner. Many children on the spectrum have strengths in nonverbal or visual processing and challenges in verbal processing; therefore, they are more likely to process pictorial representations of procedures more effectively than verbal descriptions and experience less anxiety as a result. Tools for creating a visual schedule for the doctor's visit

can be found on the Positively Autism website (www.positivelyautism.com/downloads/DoctorVisit_Story.pdf) and the Autism Speaks website (www.autismspeaks.org/tool-kit/atnair-p-visual-supports-and-autism).

- **Teach and practice calming strategies.** Teaching and practicing self-calming strategies such as doing deep breathing, listening to music, and giving deep hugs can be very helpful when the child experiences stress in a variety of situations at the clinician's office or elsewhere.
- **Encourage the family to bring items they think may be helpful for the child.** Examples include
  - Noise-canceling headphones or earplugs
  - Soothing toys or manipulatives
  - Tablet with a headset
  - Extra person to help
  - Notebook with space provided for taking notes during a visit
  - Rewards to encourage the child to try new and challenging experiences
  - Healthy snacks for encouragement and soothing
  - Comfort items, such as preferred toys or a music player

Supporting the Autistic Child During the Office Visit

There are many ways in which proactive planning by the office staff, clinicians, and parents can support a child during the pediatric visit. All children are familiar with the stress associated with this visit, but there are effective adjustments to the routines that can achieve a positive outcome. Simple adaptations include

- **Collecting feedback from parent and child about the best ways to support them during the visit:** This will help the clinician better understand what accommodations will be helpful for the family and the child.
- **Adjusting the flow of the visit:** Some children will need to have the ability to move freely rather than sit in a crowded waiting area. They might be more comfortable if allowed to wait outside the office or in a hallway, where they can play or be less restricted. To allow for this, the family may be texted when the nurse is ready to take them into an examination room.
- **Stating clearly what will happen at each step of the visit:** Many children will better understand a pictorial or visual schedule in addition to step-by-step verbal cues. Clinicians should use reinforcers and accommodations, when possible, to encourage the child and allay anxieties. Clinicians can ask the parent to bring an item or two that serve as behavioral reinforcement for the child during a procedure (eg, preferred toys, a tablet, sensory items) or can let the child know when they can have a break or access to a preferred object or activity after completing challenging tasks.

- **Demonstrating noninvasive procedures on a sibling or parent or allowing the child to learn about the equipment:** Demonstrate how the otoscope turns on and off, allow the child to inflate and deflate the blood pressure cuff, and allow them, when appropriate, to hold some of the equipment. They may learn about the examination by watching a social story or video about each step (refer to www.positivelyautism.com/downloads/DoctorVisit_Story.pdf). Suggesting that the child be given a "doctor's kit" to play with at home before a visit can enhance their understanding and acceptance of examination procedures.
- **Allowing for flexibility and extra time during each step of the examination:** Ask permission and be certain the child understands what to expect. Some children will be more comfortable if vital signs, vaccinations, and vision and hearing screenings are performed after the examination or in the examination room. Clinicians may adapt the examination to the responses of and feedback from the child.
- **Proceeding slowly and calmly while explaining each step:** These adjustments will provide the child with a sense of control.
- **Using sensory tools:** There are no uniform guidelines, but clinical experience bears out that many children on the autism spectrum seek the manipulation of sensory materials to self-calm. These materials can be effective to distract, calm, and help children on the spectrum self-regulate during a stressful experience. Clinicians can place sensory toys near the vital signs area or have parents bring familiar toys from home to provide distraction and reinforce the child's success at each step. Allow the child to play with these sensory toys. Refer to **Box 4.1** for a list of sensory tools and toys that can be beneficial in the pediatric office.

BOX 4.1 Sensory Tools and Toys to Consider for the Office

- Mirrored wall
- Wall-mounted panels with moving pictures such as video displays or moving parts such as spinning parts
- A tablet attached to the wall
- Decorative items hung from ceilings, such as model airplanes, model planets, or toy animals
- Peel-and-stick wall decals
- Light filters
- White noise machines to filter out sound
- Sensory manipulatives, such as fidget toys, balls to squeeze, games to manipulate, rainmaker toys, or bubble wands

- **Having an examination room with a lower sensory load:** The room may be set off from activity, have filtered or dimmable lighting, offer more space, contain fewer potentially anxiety-provoking or stimulating materials (visible medical equipment), and include manipulative sensory toys. Clinicians can also consider having a room without an examination table and with all instruments put away.

Goals for the Visit

- **Define goals and strengths at each visit.** By reviewing IEPs and progress notes, observing the child, and obtaining history from the parents, clinicians can facilitate discussion with families about care goals or areas to focus on. Clinicians should solicit the parents' perspective on new care goals and discuss progress and barriers to progress. It is important that the clinician have a method for documentation. (Refer to the template in Appendix A, Autism Monitoring Tool for the Pediatric Primary Care Clinician.)
- **Mark progress and celebrate successes.** Many families will benefit from articulating successes and celebrating them. This type of strength-based approach will reinforce the clinician's relationship with a family and provide encouragement and confidence to families experiencing the needs of a child on the autism spectrum. Providing encouragement is an effective tool for the pediatric clinician who is positioned to witness developmental growth in the child. When observing goals met or developmental skills mastered, clinicians should discuss these successes and proceed to discuss what logical next steps might be anticipated. For example, if a child had struggled with transition from a preferred activity and is now able to do this with support or with an incentive provided, the clinician can discuss with the family a plan for working on this type of transition in a variety of unstructured settings, such as when shopping in a grocery store or when leaving a toy section in a store, leaving playtime to come to the table, or leaving the playground. (This is discussed in more detail in Chapter 9, Autism and Behavioral Challenges: Why They Occur and How to Approach Them.)
- **Check in with family members.** Review progress at home, ways the family is adjusting, and possible needs for supports for the family.

Training Staff to Support Success at Each Visit

The nursing staff can benefit from training to understand the broad spectrum of expressions of autism and the necessity of an individualized set of accommodations to best support each child's experience in the office. The training should discuss how children on the autism spectrum may respond negatively to seemingly mundane experiences (eg, being under fluorescent lights, hearing a sudden noise, spending time in a crowded place, being touched or held, having to hold still) and how they can benefit from adjustments to the environment or routines to help them be more comfortable and better able to participate in office procedures. There may be certain predictable experiences that are particularly stressful for children on the spectrum, such as the application of a blood pressure cuff or receipt of a vaccine. There may be other triggers that are totally unexpected, such as entering a room with bright lighting or hearing a sound in the room that is inaudible to others. Staff should be educated about options for communication using the child's preferred form (eg, American Sign Language, verbal, pictorial, or a communication app) and about strategies for adapting the flow of the visit, being aware of the child's anxiety or sensory vulnerabilities, and strategies for making accommodations that have been discussed in this chapter.

The staff should have the opportunity to review the importance of bias and assumption about the ability of individuals with disabilities or neurodivergence. It is important to be aware that many individuals, including medical professionals, may make assumptions about a child's limitations or cognitive abilities and act in a way to devalue them. This behavior is a form of discrimination called *ableism,* which contributes to the inequities children on the spectrum and their families experience. The emphasis and training should be focused on assuming the child is competent and able to understand and process information from the pediatric visit but would benefit from a series of adaptations to the visit.

Billing and Coding for the Visit for the Child With Behavioral and Developmental Complexity: An Overview

The care proposed for the autistic child may require additional time before, during, and after each visit and may require special consideration for scheduling and coding. There are ways to structure longer and more complex visits, preparation for a visit, review of the EHR, report writing, and care coordination using additional *Current Procedural Terminology* (*CPT*) codes.

- Clinicians can consider scheduling a semiannual review with the parent and child or may consider scheduling more frequent visits with the child for concerns related to their developmental disability and its associated complexities and bill accordingly.
- Clinicians may code for the amount of time used to prepare for the visit by reviewing the medical record, creating orders, implementing a care plan, and planning care coordination on the day of the visit.
- If the patient visit and the time needed for record review, patient management, and care coordination extend beyond the time allotted for the preventive care or evaluation and management visit or are more than 74 minutes, clinicians can add codes for "prolonged service," "developmental testing," or "screening" as listed in **Box 4.2**.
- Clinicians can bill for time they or their staff spend engaging in chronic care management.

BOX 4.2 *Current Procedural Terminology* Codes for the Care of the Child With Medical Complexity

I. Established Patient Codes for Visits for Evaluation and Management

Time, min	Code	Medical Decision-Making
10+	**99212**	Straightforward
20+	**99213**	Low-level
30+	**99214**	Moderate
40+	**99215**	High-level
Prolonged Service		
Appointment lasting >75 minutes, 1 unit for each additional 15-minute increment	**99417**	High-level

II. Developmental Testing

- Neurobehavioral status examination without use of standardized instrument; including interpretation/report
  First hour **96116**
  Each additional hour **96121**
- Developmental screening using rating scales with scoring and documentation along with a visit
  Up to 2 per visit, must append modifier **25** to the E/M code **96110**
- Developmental testing (language, motor, cognition, social, memory, and/or executive functions) using standardized instrument; includes scoring, interpretation, and report for a visit lasting more than 30 minutes. Must append modifier **25** to the E/M code to demonstrate this was necessary to the visit.
  First hour **96112**
  Each additional 30 minutes **96113**

III. Chronic Care Coordination Services: Physician or other qualified health professional care management codes for patients with 2 or more chronic conditions expected to last at least 12 months and placing the child at significant risk for death, decline, or exacerbation. A comprehensive care plan should be documented in the electronic health record.

- Noncomplex coordination of care across providers provided by staff under physician supervision
  At least 20 minutes per month **99490**
  Additional 20 minutes per month **99439**
- Chronic care management provided by a physician or other qualified health professional
  At least 30 minutes per month **99491**
  Additional 30 minutes per month **99437**
- Complex chronic care management; moderate- or high-complexity decision-making provided by staff under the direction of a health care professional. The staff revises or establishes a comprehensive care plan.
  Up to 60 minutes per month **99487**
  Additional 30 minutes per month **99489**

Abbreviation: E/M, evaluation and management.

- The billing office should review the practice's history of collections from the different insurance providers for billing using codes for more specialized and/or lengthy visits to help inform their coding strategy.

The comprehensive care plan (as defined by the *CPT* codes) must be documented by the physician and will determine the work the staff performs. It should include the following information:

- A list of findings
- The prognosis
- Treatment goals
- Medication management
- Symptom management
- Community services used
- Plan to coordinate services
- The follow-up plan

For a more comprehensive discussion of coding, refer to the American Academy of Pediatrics coding resources (https://publications.aap.org/codingnews/info-parent/27376/Coding-Resources) or the American Medical Association 2023 guidelines (www.ama-assn.org/system/files/2023-e-m-descriptors-guidelines.pdf).

CASE VIGNETTE: CONCLUSION

The pediatrician steps into the waiting area to welcome the child and parent and recognizes the child from a prior visit. This is a young nonspeaking child who previously received a diagnosis of autism and who becomes anxious at each office visit. The clinician learns from the parent that the parent and child had been waiting for more than 30 minutes and it is now the child's nap time. The clinician understands that the child becomes anxious on entering the office and being asked to remain still in a waiting area full of people. The parent additionally describes that during a previous visit, the child became agitated when the nurse took his vital signs and pulled away when ushered back to the examination room. The parent is offered the option to reschedule the visit, but the clinician and parent decide together to resume the visit since the child is more comfortable in the quiet of the examination room.

The clinician and parent sit down for a discussion and make the following plan to support the child for more successful visits in the future:

- For future appointments, the child should be allowed to wait outside the office and then notified when the pediatrician is available so the child may be guided directly to an examination room.

Continued on next page

- The clinician and parent decide whether the first or last appointment of the day would be mutually beneficial. All attempts will be made by office staff to be punctual.
- All vital signs will be taken with a nurse trained to manage the child's anxiety.
- The parent will create or download a visual schedule to prepare the child for the visit and the two of them will practice taking vital signs and/or the parent and child will watch videos about doctor visits and taking vital signs.
- The staff and parent will support the use of sensory tools to distract the child from procedures, reinforce cooperation with procedures, and identify calming strategies the child can use when feeling stressed.
- These accommodations will be documented in an agreed-on location in the health record so the notes are visible to others working with and scheduling appointments for the child.
- The clinician will use chronic care management coding for up to 30 minutes per month outside the visit (**99491**) and each additional half hour per month (**99437**) as they review the patient's records and participate in care coordination. The staff, under the supervision of the clinician, will bill up to 60 minutes per month for complex chronic care management using the code **99487** when making or responding to follow-up phone calls. The findings, care goals, management, referrals, and follow-up plan will be documented in the child's health record. The clinician elects to bring the child back to the office at least every 6 months using established patient care codes for the high-level evaluation used to review the child's progress and screen for associated medical complexities (**99215**).

This conversation leads to a further discussion of care goals focusing on teaching the child to request a break and use strategies for self-calming. Triggers for the child's anxiety are identified, and the clinician and parent will discuss a care plan for anxiety with the child's behavioral therapist to develop more programming around exposure therapy and self-calming through everyday experiences. The parent may consider bringing the child to the office only for social visits, so he can gain some familiarity and ease with the staff.

At the end of each health supervision visit for children on the autism spectrum, it is optimal for the pediatric primary care clinician to take note of successes and challenges they experienced with the child in the office. The clinician can use this information in a collaborative fashion with the parent to better define new or revised care goals. The components of the health supervision visit that are challenging for the child are likely relevant to other responses the child has to everyday experiences and are therefore relevant to the care plan. In addition, a discussion of strategies that were successful and others that could be used in future visits should be included in the conversation with the parent. These strategies may be helpful for other children with similar developmental profiles.

Clinical Pearls

To effectively support productive office visits and positive clinical care experiences for children on the autism spectrum and their families, it is suggested that pediatric clinicians approach visits as follows:

- Identify children who may struggle at a visit. The scheduling staff can be trained to ask questions that identify which children will benefit from accommodations with scheduling and aspects of the examination.
- Plan proactively. Optimally, the practice will put protocols into place to be certain the documents from schools and specialists are available for review. It is suggested that the office compile lists of local resources to share with families, create easy forms for electronic record documentation, and teach parents how to use strategies and tools to prepare the child for the visit.
- Be flexible with the flow of the visit. Some children will benefit from being able to remain outside the office until the clinicians are ready or from being able to have flexibility with different aspects of the process (eg, when vital signs are taken, which examination room they are placed into).
- Use visual schedules to support the child's understanding of what to expect at the visit.
- Use sensory toys to distract the child, reinforce behavior, and support self-regulation.
- Document observations of the visit to better prepare for the next visit.
- Have the child return to care more regularly (at least every 6 months) to address the clinical issues related to autism.
- Learn how to bill for the extra time involved in care management.
- Identify and use care navigators or designate staff members who can assist families with the process of navigating community resources.

References

American Academy of Pediatrics. *AAP Pediatr Coding Newsl.* 2020;16(1)

American Academy of Pediatrics. Coding for standardized assessment, screening and testing. 2023. Accessed February 26, 2026. https://downloads.aap.org/AAP/PDF/coding_factsheet_developmentalscreeningtestingandEmotionalBehvioraassessment.pdf

Weitzman C, Nadler C, Blum NJ, Augustyn M; Supporting Access for Everyone Consensus Panel. Health care for youth with neurodevelopmental disabilities: a consensus statement. *Pediatrics.* 2024;153(5):e2023063809 PMID: 38596852 doi: 10.1542/peds.2023-063809

CHAPTER

5

Autism Screening in Primary Care

CASE VIGNETTE

A family well-known to the practice schedules an appointment for their 15-month-old son. Their older son received a diagnosis of autism 3 years prior, and they are concerned by their 15-month-old's persistent and repetitive banging behavior. The child's father is a drummer, they have multiple instruments in the home, and the child experiences the father practicing his drumming. The older child has significant expressive language delay and many repetitive, sensory-seeking behaviors. The parents seek advice about the increased likelihood of autism in their younger child. The pediatric primary care clinician considers how to structure the appointment, what tools to use, and, ultimately, whether to refer the child for specialist evaluation.

All children should be systematically screened for developmental delays through a combination of surveillance, developmental screening, and autism-specific screening. This requires that clinicians use their clinical skills to monitor a child's development at each health supervision visit. The American Academy of Pediatrics (AAP) practice parameters support standardized developmental screening at 9, 18, and 30 months of age. There is no specific recommendation about which tool to use. A more complete discussion of screening tools can be found in the AAP clinical report "Promoting Optimal Development: Identifying Infants and Young Children With Developmental Disorders Through Developmental Surveillance and Screening." Many clinicians in practice will use either the Parents' Evaluation of Developmental Status (PEDS) or the Ages and Stages Questionnaire (ASQ). In addition to the use of one of these proprietary level I parent questionnaires, the AAP recommends that autism-specific screening be performed at 18 and 24 months. The use of standardized tools is imperative in detecting autism; clinical judgment can vary widely, and even skilled clinicians will miss 39% of autism diagnoses by relying on general impressions alone.

Autism-Specific Screening Tools

Autism screening tools are typically divided into level I and level II screeners. Level I screeners are used for the general population, to identify individuals with indicators of autism who have a family history of autism (siblings or parents) or those who have already been identified as having findings suggestive of a diagnosis. There are many screening tools available, but those most frequently used will be reviewed in this chapter. The tool that has rigorous psychometric data to support its use, is free to use, and is available in many languages is the Modified Checklist for Autism in Toddlers, Revised with Follow-Up (M-CHAT-R/F). The M-CHAT-R/F screener is a copyrighted 20-item, 2-part parent questionnaire that is available as a free download (www.mchatscreen.com). Although this tool has many strengths and is frequently used by clinicians, its limitations are reviewed later in this chapter. It may be used for children 16 to 30 months of age to determine whether a child has indicators of autism. The initial questionnaire is completed by a parent or caregiver before or at a health supervision visit, and children with a low-likelihood score of 2 or less should be screened again at a subsequent visit if the child is 24 months or younger when first screened. If areas of concern or atypicality are revealed through screening or surveillance, children should be evaluated further and followed closely regardless of the low-likelihood screening results. If the child's score is between 3 and 7, the clinician should administer the follow-up interview to the caregiver to clarify positive responses for greater positive predictive value. A persistent score of 2 or greater on the follow-up interview indicates a high likelihood of autism. In this context, an autism diagnostic evaluation is suggested. For children with a high-likelihood score of greater than 8 at initial screening, further investigation or referral for a possible autism diagnosis should take place without the need for the follow-up interview. **Figure 5.1** shows an algorithm for determining the need for further evaluation based on a child's M-CHAT-R/F score.

Of the initial medium-likelihood positive M-CHAT-R/F scores, 36.8% will remain positive on the follow-up interview. When children whose scores remained positive were referred for evaluation, 95% met criteria for a variety of developmental challenges, but only 48% received a specific autism diagnosis. Of the children whose scores remained positive on the follow-up interview, 5% were classified as typically developing. The tool is therefore sensitive and valid for developmental disabilities but is not highly specific for autism. Children identified by the M-CHAT-R/F as having a medium likelihood of autism, but not meeting diagnostic criteria for autism, require ongoing monitoring, as they are likely to later be identified as having related developmental challenges. The M-CHAT-R/F, therefore, is able to identify children with autism indicators at earlier ages than when clinical impression or parental report alone is used.

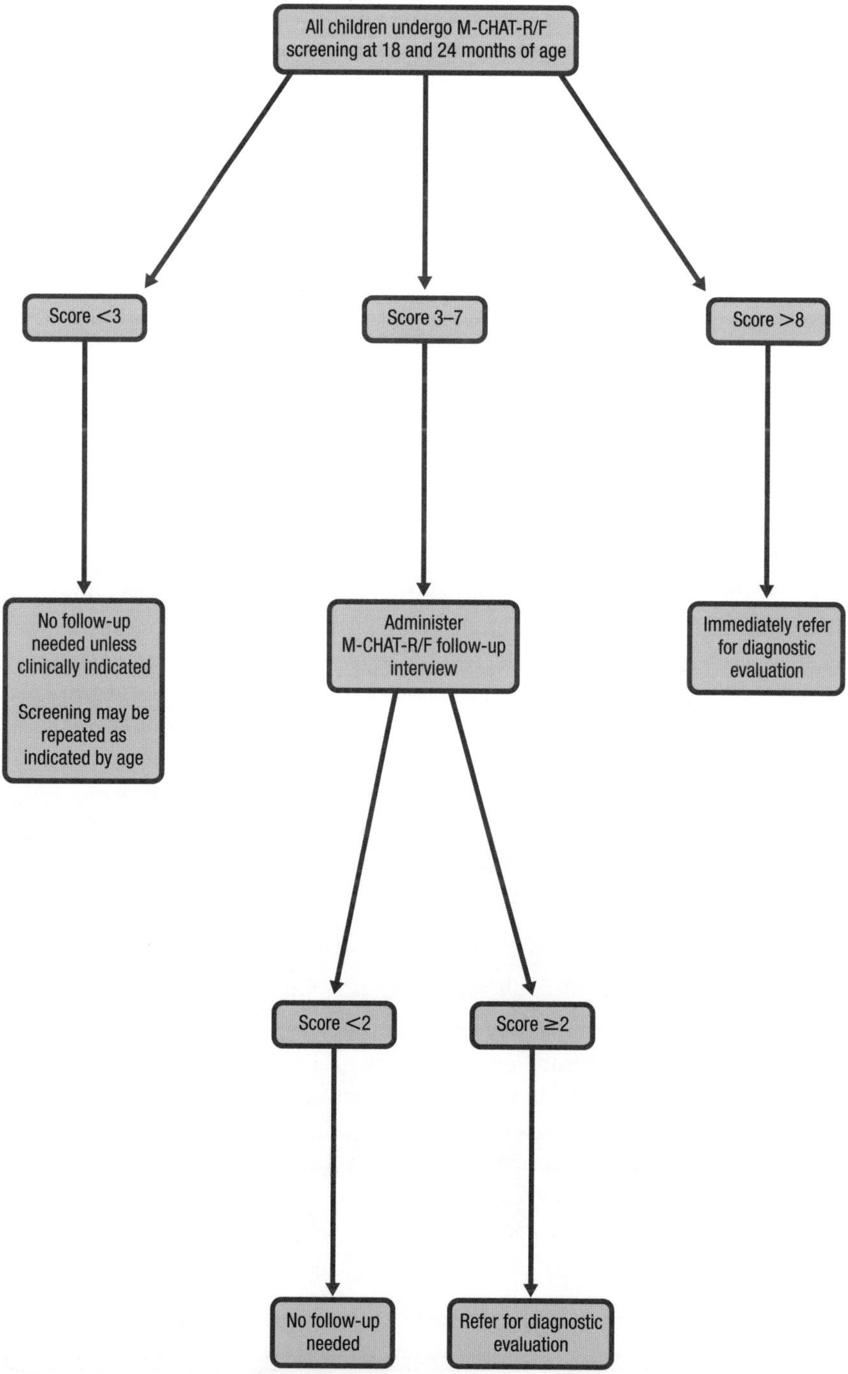

Figure 5.1. Algorithm for Evaluation of Children Based on Modified Checklist for Autism in Toddlers, Revised with Follow-Up (M-CHAT-R/F) Score

Reporting of autism indicators varies across cultures; therefore, the M-CHAT-R/F screener may be less reliable in some cultural settings. The research data on autism identification are heavily skewed toward high-income groups in Western cultures. In low-income countries, autism screening tools seem to have low sensitivity and many children remain unidentified, so there are little available supports and services. Although the domains affected in autism remain consistent across cultures, qualitative differences exist based on cultural tendencies. The most consistently reliable features of autism are delays in joint attention, communication, and social engagement, whereas the atypical features of restricted and repetitive behaviors are less consistently reported across all cultures. In some cultures, eye contact is not a social norm that is encouraged; therefore, concerns related to eye contact are likely to be reported less often. The reported effects of autism expressions may vary across cultures, or specific behaviors thought not to be indicative of autism, such as initiation of greeting others, may be heavily practiced and be present in the face of delays in joint attention. There is a great need for further research and the development of culturally sensitive tools for assessment and therapy for global use.

There are other level I parent questionnaires that can be used to screen children for autism (**Table 5.1**). Most can be completed by a caregiver and/or a teacher (when available). These questionnaires can be used to identify indicators of possible autism as well as areas of challenge that require therapy. The level II screeners are used for children already identified as having an increased likelihood (eg, siblings of those already identified or those with high-likelihood level I screening results) and involve clinician training and administration (**Table 5.1**). Some are nonproprietary and free to use, while others require registration, training, and a payment for the tool. The psychometric properties are also listed in **Table 5.1**.

The Need to Identify Concerns Early

Pediatric clinicians are often torn between the need to explore concerns and reassure parents. It is natural to rely on reassurance, especially in situations where there is uncertainty or there are few effective supports and services to offer. In the case of autism, however, clinicians have an opportunity to refer the child when concern is identified during the early months of critical development. Research clearly supports the efficacy of early intervention (EI); therefore, referrals need to be made as expeditiously as possible to allow for early developmental support. This is discussed in more detail in Chapter 8, Evidence-Based Supports and Services.

Table 5.1. Autism Screening Tools

Screening Tool	Time to Administer, min	Type	Age Range	Sensitivity, %	Specificity, %
Level I Screeners to Identify Likelihood of Autism					
Autism Spectrum Rating Scales (ASRS) Available at www.pearsonassessments.com	15–20	Parent/teacher rating	2–18 y	89.8–95[a]	90.3–94.7[a]
Childhood Autism Spectrum Test (CAST) Available at www.autismresearchcentre.com/tests/childhood-autism-spectrum-test-cast	20	Parent rating	4–11 y	100[b]	97[b]
Communication and Symbolic Behavior Scales Developmental Profile Infant-Toddler Checklist (CSBS DP ITC) Free at https://brookespublishing.com/resource-library/csbs-dp-infant-toddler-checklist/	10	Parent rating	6–24 mo	94[c]	88.9[c]
Modified Checklist for Autism in Toddlers, Revised with Follow-Up (M-CHAT-R/F) Free at www.mchatscreen.com	5	Parent rating	16–30 mo	82.6[d]	45.7 with follow-up interview[d]
Social Communication Questionnaire (SCQ) Available at www.wpspublish.com	10	Parent rating	4+ y	93[e]	58[e]
Social Responsiveness Scale, Second Edition (SRS-2) Available at www.wpspublish.com	15–20	Parent/teacher rating	2.5–18 y	96[f]	95[f]
The Survey of Well-being of Young Children (SWYC) Free at www.teamupcenter.org/swyc	5	Parent rating	16–35 mo	89[g]	56[g]

Continued on next page

Table 5.1 *(continued)*

Screening Tool	Time to Administer, min	Type	Age Range	Sensitivity, %	Specificity, %
Level II Screeners for Children Already Identified as Having an Increased Likelihood of Autism					
Rapid Interactive Screening Test for Autism in Toddlers (RITA-T) Requires training and tools Online training available at www.kennedykrieger.org/research/centers-labs-cores/rita-t-research	10	Direct administration	18–36 mo	100[h]	84[h]
Screening Tool for Autism in Toddlers and Young Children (STAT) Requires training and tools Available at https://vkc.vumc.org/vkc/triad/stat Remote version available at https://triad.vkclearning.org/en-us	20	Direct administration	24–36 mo	92[i]	85[i]

[a] Goldstein S, Naglieri JA. *Autism Spectrum Rating Scales (ASRS) Technical Report #2:* DSM-5 *Update.* Multi-Health Systems; 2014.

Camodeca A. Description of criterion validity of the Autism Spectrum Rating Scales 6–18 parent report: initial exploration in a large community sample. *Child Psychiatry Hum Dev.* 2019;50(6):987–1001.

[b] Williams J, Scott F, Stott C, et al. The CAST (Childhood Asperger Syndrome Test): test accuracy. *Autism.* 2005;9(1):45–68.

[c] Wetherby AM, Allen L, Cleary J, Kublin K, Goldstein H. Validity and reliability of the Communication and Symbolic Behavior Scales Developmental Profile with very young children. *J Speech Lang Hear Res.* 2002;45(6):1202–1218.

[d] Aishworiya R, Ma VK, Stewart S, Hagerman R, Feldman HM. Meta-analysis of the Modified Checklist for Autism in Toddlers, Revised/Follow-Up for screening. *Pediatrics.* 2023;151(6):e2022059393.

[e] Nguyen PH, Ocansey ME, Miller M, Le DTK, Schmidt RJ, Prado EL. The reliability and validity of the Social Responsiveness Scale to measure autism symptomology in Vietnamese children. *Autism Res.* 2019;12(11):1706–1718.

[f] Constantino JN, Davis SA, Todd RD, et al. Validation of a brief quantitative measure of autistic traits: comparison of the Social Responsiveness Scale with the Autism Diagnostic Interview-Revised. *J Autism Dev Disord.* 2003;33(4):427–433.

[g] Lipkin PH, Macias MM; American Academy of Pediatrics Council on Children With Disabilities and Section on Developmental and Behavioral Pediatrics. Promoting optimal development: identifying infants and young children with developmental disorders through developmental surveillance and screening. *Pediatrics.* 2020;145(1):e20193449.

[h] Kong XJ, Sherman HT, Tian R, et al. Validation of Rapid Interactive Screening Test for Autism in Toddlers using Autism Diagnostic Observation Schedule Second Edition in children at high-risk for autism spectrum disorder. *Front Psychiatry.* 2021;12:737890.

[i] Stone WL, Coonrod EE, Turner LM, Pozdol SL. Psychometric properties of the STAT for early autism screening. *J Autism Dev Disord.* 2004;34(6):691–701.

As in this chapter's opening case, the clinician has a choice to consider a primary care evaluation with either certain or provisional diagnosis or to refer the child for a full neuropsychological evaluation. Because there may be benefit from the early introduction of support, referrals are recommended even for subthreshold clinical concern. What is needed in the case vignette is a systematic review of likelihood, an understanding of the tools available, and an organized approach to assessing likelihood while the child and parent are present.

Taking Time to Observe and Categorize Behavior

When a child has been identified as having an increased likelihood of autism, the clinician should have a system for making and documenting developmental observations to assess whether a diagnosis of autism is to be considered. Some clinicians will choose to obtain specific training to make a diagnosis by using level II screeners (refer to Chapter 6, Establishing the Autism Diagnosis, for more details); others will simply use a systematic approach to organizing behaviors indicative of autism elicited from the child's history and a qualitative observation in the office.

There are multiple methods a clinician can use to capitalize on time with the child to identify possible indicators of autism and whether further evaluation or referral is relevant. This information can aid the clinician in interpreting parent reports or results of formal standardized screening as decisions are made for next steps in assessment and support. It is important to take advantage of opportunities to observe the child, elicit developmental strengths, and identify possible concerns around atypical features and to implement a system for categorizing observations. Clinicians should take a few minutes to either observe the child with the caregiver or sit on the floor with the child if able and create opportunities for observation of the following skills:

- **Social play:** Collect toys such as bubbles, a toy car, or a ball made from examination table paper, or play a game of drumming on the table, to initiate and observe the child in back-and-forth play. Roll or toss the toy back and forth. Blow the bubbles using a machine/bubble blower or flick of the wand to alleviate concerns about spreading germs. After initiating any play, stop and wait to observe how the child communicates with the adult to make a request to resume play. Avoid giving a verbal instruction or directing the child; simply sit and observe the child's responses. Note whether and how the child uses eye contact, pointing, and words. Sit and wait or make a gesture, such as putting your hands up to indicate waiting for the toy to be passed or for the child to imitate your behaviors. Repeat the actions to see if you can elicit multiple turns in back-and-forth play and requests for "more."

- **Imitation:** Model a new action such as putting blocks into a horizontal chain and pretending it is a train. Make the "choo choo" sound of a train to get the child's attention, then take apart the train and hand the blocks to the child. Instruct the child to build the train using a phrase such as "Now, you do it." Observe if the child is able to imitate a new action. Consider asking the parent to model the new action if the child does not respond.
- **Pretend play:** Watch the child while taking breaks in between the components of the examination or while talking with the caregiver. Put a few toys onto the floor and observe how the child plays: Do they explore in a sensory-based fashion by simply touching, arranging, looking, banging, mouthing, or pushing, or do they use toys in an appropriate and varied fashion? Introduce an idea into the play (eg, feeding or rocking a baby) or have the parent do this. Model pretend play by engaging in an action such as parking a toy car, having the car "go to school," or providing a pretend snack to a doll or figure. Introduce a conversation or a symbolic action such as eating or sleeping. Alternatively, play in parallel with the child and have your toy or object converse or interact with theirs.
- **Attachment behavior:** Observe how the child interacts with the parent or uses communication skills to express anxiety and seek relief and comfort from the parent. This may indicate whether there is secure attachment. Watch to see if the child will share with the parent or initiate play with them. Observe if the child watches the parent and seeks eye contact.
- **Response to verbal instructions:** Give a few simple instructions (eg, "Go get..." or "Where is the..."). Make these instructions about things in which the child is interested and without using pointing.
- **Unstructured play:** Allow the child the opportunity to initiate and to pursue their own interests in play while the adults sit back and only watch. This is when pretend play, exploration, social initiation, and social communication may occur. In a child on the autism spectrum, this might be the first time the examiner will observe expressions of atypicality. At this time, when there is no structure, a child might withdraw and engage in self-soothing actions or repetitive behaviors. Parents can be uncomfortable observing these behaviors without intervening, but without this unstructured time, the examiner might not have the opportunity to observe behaviors indicative of autism. This can provide a teaching moment to share with the parent the observations of the child's behavior that may warrant further investigation and possible support.
- **At home:** Consider having the parent/caregiver share home videos. Ask for videos demonstrating both concerns around atypical behaviors and areas of strength.

Once the clinician has developed a method for collecting more information and observing the child, a system for documenting these observations is helpful. Many clinicians will use a checklist based on the *Diagnostic and Statistical Manual of Mental Disorders, Fifth Edition, Text Revision* criteria or an elaborated checklist of behaviors that fit into the diagnostic criteria, as shown in **Box 5.1**. These checklists

BOX 5.1 Checklist of Characteristics Suggestive of Autism

A. Speech and sounds

- ☐ Absence of words or word approximations
- ☐ Use of speech sounds that narrate or label and are not directed to a person
- ☐ Absence of language to make requests
- ☐ Not sharing enjoyment
- ☐ Not using language to draw the attention of others (eg, “Look,” “See”)
- ☐ Absence of back-and-forth use of language
- ☐ Atypical nonword noises
- ☐ Atypical intonation

B. Coordinating eye contact/gestures/speech or vocalizations

- ☐ Absence or paucity of gesture use (eg, pointing, reaching, clapping, beckoning)
- ☐ Inability to coordinate eye contact with gesture use or vocalization
- ☐ Use of caregiver’s hand as a tool to seek access to what is desired

C. Play

- ☐ Only functional play present (eg, pushing a car, putting a doll into a chair)
- ☐ Lack or paucity of pretend play
- ☐ Difficulty imitating
- ☐ Repetitive or unusual play (eg, lining up objects, scrambling/dropping/throwing toys)
- ☐ Preoccupation with a certain toy/activity

D. Body movements

- ☐ Hand flapping
- ☐ Posturing
- ☐ Tensing of body
- ☐ Toe walking
- ☐ Facial grimacing
- ☐ Hand/finger mannerisms
- ☐ Repetitive running/walking/spinning/bouncing/jumping

E. Sensory differences

- ☐ Visual inspection
- ☐ Seeking out textures or tight spaces
- ☐ Mouthing/licking objects
- ☐ Sound/light/texture sensitivity
- ☐ Self-injury (eg, scratching or biting self, head banging)
- ☐ Noise sensitivity

Adapted from Vanderbilt University Medical Center. Autism Interview for Caregivers of Young Children. Vanderbilt Kennedy Center. Accessed February 26, 2026. https://vkc.vumc.org.

may be used to organize observations or to make a provisional diagnosis, as discussed in Chapter 6, Establishing the Autism Diagnosis, or document indicators suggestive of a diagnosis. Many clinicians are becoming more actively involved in assessment and referral for therapy. Although the AAP and most specialists advocate for the use of standardized level II screeners, some insurance companies may acknowledge a provisional diagnosis once the observations are well described and organized. Unfortunately, many insurance providers have rules about which diagnostic tools to use despite the fact that the literature does not give priority to one method of diagnosis over another.

Clinicians should consider obtaining training for selected autism diagnosis in primary care. Refer to Chapter 6, Establishing the Autism Diagnosis, for more information about the pediatric primary care clinician and triaging diagnosis.

Early Referral for the Child Identified as Having an Increased Likelihood of Autism

Many families will wait for months or years to receive a comprehensive developmental evaluation and a definitive diagnosis of autism. The specific concerns of the clinician should be discussed with the parent as soon as possible. Refer to Chapter 6, Establishing the Autism Diagnosis, for a more thorough discussion of sharing concerns and a diagnosis with a parent. In the interim, it is imperative that guidance is provided to the parent to support an optimal developmental course while the family is awaiting a developmental and autism evaluation. The clinician should consider scheduling time with the parent to review the identified concerns. This review is an opportunity for the clinician to make specific recommendations to the parent about how to work on play and engagement at home and to refer for specific supports and services even before a conclusive diagnosis has been made. Materials for parents are available to guide this work, and it is helpful for clinicians to have resource lists for their region to share, including lists of specialists and allied health professionals. **Box 5.2** lists recommendations for materials and resources to share with parents while families are awaiting a diagnosis.

BOX 5.2 How the Primary Care Clinician Can Support Families While They Are Awaiting an Autism Evaluation

- Explain specific concerns and the importance of early and evidence-based support. Provide the family with the following resources to learn more about autism:
  - Autism Speaks: www.autismspeaks.org
  - HealthyChildren.org, the official American Academy of Pediatrics website for parents, "Understanding Autism: Information for Families": www.healthychildren.org/English/health-issues/conditions/Autism/Pages/Autism-Spectrum-Disorder.aspx
- Identify specific areas of concern that can be addressed immediately.
- Refer for early intervention and a diagnostic evaluation.
- Consider assigning a nurse administrator in the practice to follow up with and support the family in this process. Identify members of the practice who can compile lists of local resources for a child on the autism spectrum, perhaps a summer intern or medical student.
- Refer the child for appropriate private therapies (speech, occupational, and/or behavioral).
- Give guidance when relevant to support engagement and joint attention. For parent guidance on promoting skills of engagement, refer to the following resources:
  - The Hanen Centre: www.hanen.org/information-tips/autism
  - The Early Start Denver Model: www.esdm.co
  - Help is in Your Hands: www.helpisinyourhands.org (free registration required)
  - The section How can I support my child? in Appendix B, Parent Handout: What Is Autism and How Do I Know if My Preschool-Aged Child Is on the Spectrum?
- Teach parents to emphasize on-the-floor, face-to-face, back-and-forth play and engagement. Advise that they avoid teaching skills that promote the rote recitation or repetitive teaching of early academic skills (the alphabet, shapes, colors, or phonics) or relying on electronic toys to "teach" skills.
- Advise parents to remove electronic toys and interact, take turns, and follow the child's lead in play.
- Suggest basic behavioral strategies such as introducing predictable routines and structure, using visual aids, and distracting and redirecting for dysregulated behavior, as discussed on the Lives in the Balance website at https://livesinthebalance.org/parents-and-families-tour.
- Evaluate for associated difficulties with sleep, exercise, eating and nutrition, sensory processing, and behavioral challenges and refer/develop care plans for each area of concern.

CASE VIGNETTE: CONCLUSION

At the health supervision visit, the pediatric primary care clinician spends an additional 10 minutes with the parents face-to-face to elicit their concerns. The clinician administers the Communication and Symbolic Behavior Scales to the parents since the 15-month-old child's age falls below the age range for administration of the M-CHAT-R/F or a level II screener. The results are not in a concerning range. The clinician uses the Checklist of Characteristics Suggestive of Autism (refer to **Box 5.1**) to systematically organize observations of the child. He learns that this child uses reach, points, and grunts to ask for help or obtain things that are out of reach. The child is noted to turn when called, brings his toys to show and share with his parents, and understands and responds to a few simple verbal instructions. His eye contact has always been discernible, and he seems to monitor and follow what his parents are engaged in. The child does not have any specific words but uses some word approximations to draw attention. The child is observed sitting with one of the parents on the floor and passing a ball back and forth while imitating the actions the parent models in play and looks up to smile with the parent. There are no atypical or stereotypical behaviors observed.

The clinician feels comfortable reassuring the parents that the child is developing appropriately and has strong skills of joint attention. This child has an increased likelihood of autism given the family history, and the clinician is aware that the repetitive and atypical features suggestive of autism may evolve as the child ages. The clinician provides the parents with a resource on supporting play skills and recommends a return visit within 3 months to administer the M-CHAT-R/F or a level II screener at 18 months of age and general developmental screening and follow-up with the parents. The clinician does not feel referrals are indicated at this time, and the parents are reassured.

Clinical Pearls

- Autism-specific standardized screening tools are recommended at 18 and 24 months of age.
- All children with any concerning clinical features should be followed closely by the pediatric primary care clinician.
- When children have an increased likelihood identified by screening, the results should be reviewed verbally with the parent. It is recommended that the M-CHAT-R/F follow-up interview be used for children with intermediate scores.
- All children with identified delays and atypical features indicative of autism should be referred for EI services without waiting for a diagnostic evaluation.
- Pediatric clinicians should use clinical observation skills to further assess and document developmental concerns.
- All children identified as having a significant likelihood of autism should undergo diagnostic evaluations as soon as possible.

References

Aishworiya R, Ma VK, Stewart S, Hagerman R, Feldman HM. Meta-analysis of the Modified Checklist for Autism in Toddlers, Revised/Follow-Up for Screening. *Pediatrics.* 2023;151(6):e2022059393 PMID: 37203373 doi: 10.1542/peds.2022-059393

American Academy of Pediatrics Council on Children With Disabilities, Section on Developmental Behavioral Pediatrics, Bright Futures Steering Committee, and Medical Home Initiatives for Children With Special Needs Project Advisory Committee. Identifying infants and young children with developmental disorders in the medical home: an algorithm for developmental surveillance and screening. *Pediatrics.* 2006;118(1):405–420 PMID: 16818591 doi: 10.1542/peds.2006-1231

de Leeuw A, Happé F, Hoekstra RA. A conceptual framework for understanding the cultural and contextual factors on autism across the globe. *Autism Res.* 2020;13(7):1029–1050 PMID: 32083402 doi: 10.1002/aur.2276

Hyman SL, Levy SE, Myers SM, et al; American Academy of Pediatrics Council on Children With Disabilities and Section on Developmental and Behavioral Pediatrics. Identification, evaluation, and management of children with autism spectrum disorder. *Pediatrics.* 2020;145(1):e20193447 PMID: 31843864 doi: 10.1542/peds.2019-3447

Levy SE, Wolfe A, Coury D, et al. Screening tools for autism spectrum disorder in primary care: a systematic evidence review. *Pediatrics.* 2020;145(suppl 1):S47–S59 PMID: 32238531 doi: 10.1542/peds.2019-1895H

Lipkin PH, Macias MM; American Academy of Pediatrics Council on Children With Disabilities and Section on Developmental and Behavioral Pediatrics. Promoting optimal development: identifying infants and young children with developmental disorders through developmental surveillance and screening. *Pediatrics.* 2020;145(1):e20193449 PMID: 31843861 doi: 10.1542/peds.2019-3449

McDougle C, ed. *Autism Spectrum Disorder.* Oxford University Press; 2015 doi: 10.1093/med/9780199349722.001.0001

Robins DL, Casagrande K, Barton M, Chen CM, Dumont-Mathieu T, Fein D. Validation of the Modified Checklist for Autism in Toddlers, Revised with Follow-Up (M-CHAT-R/F). *Pediatrics.* 2014;133(1):37–45 PMID: 24366990 doi: 10.1542/peds.2013-1813

Stevanovic D, Robins DL, Costanzo F, et al. Cross-cultural similarities and differences in reporting autistic symptoms in toddlers: a study synthesizing M-CHAT(-R) data from ten countries. *Res Autism Spectr Disord.* 2022;95:101984 doi: 10.1016/j.rasd.2022.101984

CHAPTER

6

Establishing the Autism Diagnosis

CASE VIGNETTE

Jonah is a 3-year-old who presents for his health supervision appointment with a clinician he has not seen previously. This clinician notes that in addition to having expressive language delay, Jonah does not follow verbal instructions and tends to play alone. He becomes absorbed in repeatedly arranging letter sets in alphabetical order while humming the alphabet song. Jonah follows through with the examination but does not initiate interaction or visually attend to his mother or father or the clinician. When the nurse attempts to take his vital signs, Jonah begins to cry, becomes agitated, and tries to leave.

Jonah had scored in the high-likelihood range (>8) on his Modified Checklist for Autism in Toddlers, Revised with Follow-Up (M-CHAT-R/F), screening at 2 years of age and was referred for an autism evaluation by a different clinician. At the time of this 3-year appointment, he is still waiting for this evaluation. The pediatric primary care clinician is aware that there is a high likelihood of autism and that a year of opportunity for support has passed while the family waits for a specialty evaluation. The primary care clinician reviews with Jonah's parents the concerns about Jonah's developmental delays and cognitive strengths, as well as the presence of restricted and repetitive behaviors that appear to be affecting his development.

The diagnosis of autism can be made when an individual presents with a behavioral profile that meets diagnostic criteria that are not better attributed to global developmental delay or intellectual disability (ID). This diagnosis can be made by a variety of clinician types and through a variety of diagnostic tools but should be made within the context of a complete history, developmental assessment, and physical examination. A diagnosis should be made by using a combination of rating scales administered to parents and, possibly, teachers and/or caregivers;

detailed parent interview; and structured behavioral observations. Most clinicians use a variety of standardized tools for each of these diagnostic components.

Autism is a neurodevelopmental condition that must be present in the early developmental period. Autism may present later, when the demands of the environment exceed the abilities of the individual. Many of the features found in individuals on the spectrum are also found in neurotypically developing individuals, but the distinguishing feature of a diagnosis is when the characteristics or traits of autism create significant difficulties and negatively affect the child's developmental process. It is also important to understand that language delay is not a necessary criterion for diagnosis. In fact, many children on the spectrum have large vocabularies and linguistic strengths that are limited in their use within social contexts. These linguistic strengths may be related to the child's interests and strong cognitive ability to build vocabulary.

Meeting *DSM-5-TR* Diagnostic Criteria

The formal diagnosis of autism spectrum disorder is made when findings from the review of history and assessment of the child meet the diagnostic criteria as articulated in the *DSM-5-TR*. Children on the autism spectrum present with a combination of difficulties in social engagement, reciprocity, and nonverbal communication and a variety of atypical, repetitive, and/or restricted patterns of behavior and interests. The *DSM-5-TR* creates categories of characteristics and traits for securing the diagnosis. The following list includes clinical features that fit into the *DSM* diagnostic criteria:

1. **Social communication and social interaction:** The first set of criteria entail difficulties with communicative behaviors and social interaction. To qualify for a diagnosis, the child **must meet all 3 criteria in this category.**

   A. **Social-emotional reciprocity:** This relates to a child's decreased ability to initiate or respond to social interaction, decreased ability to interact in a back-and-forth manner, and decreased tendency to share interests or emotions.
   Examples:
   - Does not bring things to show or share
   - Has limited ability to initiate interaction or conversation
   - Does not ask for help
   - Struggles to make requests
   - Shares desires or excitement infrequently
   - Exhibits inconsistent responses to being given verbal instructions or being called by name
   - Tends to not respond when others invite them to play or interact

- Has limited conversational exchange
- Makes limited verbal comments

B. **Atypical nonverbal social behavior:** Children on the spectrum may not use gesture, facial expression, and eye contact for social interaction and communication as seen in other children their age. Additionally, they may not respond to the nonverbal communicative efforts of others.
Examples:
- Rarely points to show interests, direct the attention of others, or make requests
- May pull parent or hand of parent as a tool rather than use words or gesture
- Has limited gesture use (eg, shaking head, waving, putting hands up, nodding, pointing)
- Has limited use of facial expression

C. **Difficulties in maintaining relationships:** Children on the spectrum may show little interest in peers, peer play, imaginative play, or interactive play. They may not appear to understand the social rules or to modify their behavior to fit the social norms.
Examples:
- Plays alone
- Does not form close friends or interact with peers
- Tends not to join group activities
- Struggles to match behavior to the setting
- Runs from the group, engages in unsafe behavior or behavior that is disruptive to one's functioning and others' space
- Tends to engage in repetitive play, with few imaginative or turn-taking games
- Lack of response to the social invitation of others

2. **Restricted, repetitive patterns of behavior, actions, or interests:** The second set of criteria include a variety of behaviors that are unusual and not expected for children developing typically. They tend to interfere with the child's ability to meet the demands of their world by presenting as inflexibility and resulting in the child not developing the variety of skills as expected for age. To qualify for a diagnosis of autism, the child must meet criteria for **at least 2** of these 4 groups of behaviors.

A. **Stereotypical, repetitive, and/or idiosyncratic speech; motor stereotypies; or repetitive use of objects:** Children on the spectrum may demonstrate the persistent echoing of vocalizations. They may repeat what others say, may repeat rather than respond to others, or may use language they have heard or learned out of context or in an undirected fashion. They may engage in repetitive motor actions or use objects in an excessively repetitive fashion.

Examples:

- Echoes what others say.
- Echoes a question rather than responds.
- Repeats a question with pronouns reversed to respond. For example, the parent asks, "Do you want a cookie?" and the child responds, "You want a cookie?" when indicating they want a cookie.
- Repeats phrases or quotes, especially from books, videos, or things others have said.
- Uses language they have learned in a related but not totally natural manner. For example, the parent asks, "Are you tired?" and the child responds, "Ernie says I'm sleepy!"
- Displays repetitive motor stereotypies such as hand flapping, toe walking, rocking, spinning, or flicking.
- Engages in repetitive use of objects in lieu of using them as intended (eg, stacking, dropping, spinning, or examining objects; lining objects up or arranging them in a specific manner rather than playing with them in a symbolic or novel manner).

B. **Excessive adherence to routines or rituals:** These behaviors occur repeatedly and interfere with the child completing tasks, transitions, or other age-appropriate actions. The behaviors may be based on a sensory need. Children may insist on things being done, organized, and said in a specific and repetitive manner and may become distressed if routines are changed.

Examples:

- Insists on the ordering of actions, interactions, speech, and/or objects
- May become upset if the order they create with objects or actions is changed
- Insists on turning lights on and off or opening and closing doors in a specific manner
- Plays with toys in a specific and repetitive manner (eg, arranging them; lining them up by size, color, or shape)
- Struggles with change, such as new experiences or changes related to food items, driving routes, or clothing
- Has extreme behavioral responses to change

C. **Atypical sensory behavior:** Individuals on the spectrum can have unusual sensory needs. They may respond or react to low levels of sensory material (hypersensitivity) or not respond when it is expected they would (hyposensitivity). Some seek out sensory input and others may show aversion to it. Their sensitivities may be very focused on and specific to one type of sensory experience or to many. A sensitivity may be relevant to touch, visual phenomena, sounds, smells, textures, movement, and/or food.
   Examples:
   - Mouths or eats nonfood items
   - Engages in specific visual inspection, such as holding something up to the face, lying down to examine something visually, or moving back and forth to look at patterns
   - Displays hypersensitivity to certain sounds
   - Has a high pain threshold
   - Insists on food being presented in a certain manner, such as different foods not touching one another, or only tolerates foods that are of one color or texture
   - Is unable to tolerate certain sensory experiences, such as toothbrushing, hair brushing, hugs, public bathrooms, hand driers, toilet flushers, or other sounds
   - Seeks out other sensory experiences; may squeeze into tight places, make loud noises, watch light through the blinds, or activate a sound repeatedly
   - Has a limited repertoire of foods tolerated

D. **Focused interests:** The child may have a certain number of interests that may be focused in nature; therefore, the child may engage in a narrow range of activities. They may have a limited repertoire of play actions and insist on maintaining this. They may have a persistent interest in learning and talking about one topic excessively to others. (Note that this interest in certain topics can be age appropriate but will tend to vary and be less persistent.)
   Examples:
   - Has an interest in one topic, such as space, cars, trains, or dinosaurs
   - Always builds the same arrangement with blocks
   - Has an interest in letters, numbers, colors, or shapes to the exclusion of a varied amount of interests and can be distracted by their presence in the environment
   - Is interested in figuring out how things work rather than playing with them; may take things apart rather than play with them

The *DSM-5-TR* specifies that these characteristics and traits of autism must create significant challenges for the child. These challenges are essential to making the diagnosis. Children on the spectrum tend to struggle to make friends, meet requests, transition, and engage in group activities and tend to have significant difficulties in everyday skills of independence. These skills, or *activities of daily living,* refer to the ability to dress oneself, maintain hygiene as expected for age, follow rules of safety, and live independently at one's developmental level. The *DSM-5-TR* states that the characteristics and traits of autism are not explained by an ID or a global developmental delay. Although autism and ID may often coexist, it is important to understand that many individuals with ID will have atypical features or characteristics of autism. To make the diagnosis of autism, the child's social communication skills and general ability to engage socially must be more affected than would be expected for their developmental level.

In summary, the *DSM-5-TR* states that the following conditions should be specified if occurring along with the diagnosis of autism:

- Accompanying ID
- Accompanying language difficulty
- An associated genetic disorder or other developmental or mental health condition

To gain more familiarity with the presentations of autism in younger children, video can be an invaluable teaching tool. Teaching videos that provide video examples of the characteristics described in this section are available through Autism Navigator (https://autismnavigator.com/asd-video-glossary). These resources require free registration by the participant.

A Word on Severity Ratings

The *DSM-5-TR* provides guidance for determining severity ratings for a child's autism. These are based on the level of support that is required for the child to be able to engage with and respond to others in their environment and the degree of difficulty that results from the restricted and repetitive behaviors and interests. These severity ratings will vary over time and depend on the demands of different settings (home, school, and community). These levels are defined as follows:

- Level 1: requiring support
- Level 2: requiring substantial support
- Level 3: requiring very substantial support

In the young child, an assignment of a severity rating can be very confusing to parents and has not been documented to have any predictive value. One child may show tremendous improvement over a short period, and others may show more signs of difficulty if coexisting conditions present further challenges to the child's ability to progress and adapt to the demands of the environment. Further, with most young children on the autism spectrum, an intensive program with substantial support is often preferred to allow for optimal developmental progress in the early years. It is important for parents to understand that this level of intensive support is targeted toward optimizing the child's developmental course and is **not** necessarily a predictor of poor outcome. Many clinicians elect to avoid severity ratings during the preschool period unless requested by insurance providers or for school-based support.

The Potential Role of the Pediatric Primary Care Clinician in Diagnosis

Given the rising number of children affected by autism, the long wait lists for appointments, and logistical and financial barriers to obtaining care provided by subspecialty clinics, many primary care clinicians are seeking training to make autism diagnoses. A multidisciplinary assessment is not always necessary or feasible. Primary care clinicians can accurately make reliable diagnoses in approximately two-thirds of preschoolers after autism training and short-term supervision for reliability. Published research reveals agreement in diagnosis validity between the trained primary care clinicians and expert specialists in 74% to 100% of patients in well-established training programs that provide short-term supervision.

Many academic centers or state-sponsored programs across the country, such as the Virginia Mental Health Access Program (https://vmap.org), Extension for Community Healthcare Outcomes (ECHO) Autism Communities (https://echoautism.org/about-us), Children's National Center for Autism Spectrum Disorders (www.childrensnational.org/get-care/departments/center-for-autism-spectrum-disorders/provider-resources), and Kennedy Krieger Institute Rapid Interactive Screening Test for Autism in Toddlers (RITA-T) Training Course (https://rita-t.learningportal.kennedykrieger.org/courses/rita-t), provide online training and ongoing remote supervision on autism diagnostic skills for pediatric primary care clinicians in practice. This approach encourages clinicians to become involved with diagnosis and management for young children on the autism spectrum presenting with clear features and without a complexity of co-occurring conditions. It establishes a system for triage of the more complex presentations to tertiary referral centers.

In particular, ECHO Autism Communities has successfully measured the efficacy of pediatric primary care clinicians making autism diagnoses. This program has adapted the use of a Project ECHO mentoring model using videoconferencing technology. In this ECHO Autism Early Diagnosis Model, a team of experts teaches a team of local pediatric primary care clinicians through a bimonthly 90-minute brief didactic and case discussion. The model has been adapted for in-person diagnostic training followed by the addition of coaching and feedback. The program occurs over a period of a year. Outcome data from this ECHO model have demonstrated an increase in physician self-identified knowledge, resource sharing with families, and autism screening and strong reliability of use of the Screening Tool for Autism in Toddlers and Young Children (STAT), a level II diagnostic tool. The STAT, as reviewed in Chapter 5, Autism Screening in Primary Care, is a 20-minute structured assessment tool for autism in 24- to 36-month-old children that requires training and a specific tool set to administer. The STAT exists as an in-person tool and a virtual version that was developed at Vanderbilt University (TELE-ASD-PEDS). The virtual version was used successfully before and more widely during the COVID-19 pandemic. It has been particularly helpful in screening children from remote settings as well as during times when in-person assessments were not possible. The ECHO autism training has been successful in integrating pediatric primary care clinicians into autism evaluations and ongoing care. Of the pediatric primary care clinicians participating in the training, 73% reported accepting referrals for autism evaluation and 80% reported having more children on the spectrum in their practice.

Tiered Triage Model for Diagnosis

Many autism specialists now suggest a tiered approach to evaluating the young child with behaviors suggestive of autism. In this model, the primary care clinician serves to triage children with likelihood of or concern for autism, as shown in **Box 6.1**. For children with an unambiguous presentation, autism can be diagnosed by a primary care clinician, but children with a more complicated presentation should be referred for specialty evaluation with or without a diagnosis made by the primary care clinician. This model not only enables earlier and more successful diagnosis in the medical home but also allows for support during the critical early years of development, offering a greater positive effect on long-term outcomes. A secondary result of this model is to lessen the demand on the specialty centers and therefore shorten wait lists for those requiring a multispecialty evaluation.

Using Standardized Tools to Document a Diagnosis in Primary Care

If the pediatric clinician is involved in making autism diagnoses, it is imperative for both receiving insurance reimbursement and establishing care goal targets that a clinician's notes contain a thorough documentation of findings. As much as possible, it is preferable to use standardized tools that combine parent and teacher observations through rating scales, parent interview, and direct observations. Use of a checklist based on the *DSM-5-TR* criteria is helpful to demonstrate specifically and systematically how the child meets diagnostic criteria. There are several standardized questionnaires available for teachers and parents to complete that are scored and broken down into specific domains. As discussed in Chapter 5, Autism Screening in Primary Care, these questionnaires can be used, not only for population screening but also as level II screeners, to further identify the children already determined to have an increased likelihood of autism.

BOX 6.1 Pediatric Primary Care Clinician Triaging of Children With Likelihood of or Concern for Autism

Tier 1, clear characteristics of autism: In this case, the primary care clinician is readily able to make a diagnosis based on careful review of developmental history (refer to Appendix C, Sample Intake Questionnaire), clinical presentation, and physical examination without the necessary use of standardized tools. Reliance on *DSM-5-TR* checklists to ensure the child meets criteria is helpful, but it is preferable that the primary care clinician has been trained to use a standardized assessment such as the STAT. Documentation supporting *DSM-5-TR* criteria, parent interview, and a standardized behavioral observation (eg, the STAT) is helpful in insurance reimbursement and therapy initiation. Insurance companies may mandate the use of specific tools, and the primary care clinician may be called on to carefully document their findings and appeal the insurance company decisions to deny reimbursement of therapy based on the diagnosis made in primary care.

Tier 2, subtler characteristics of autism: These cases are associated with a more complicated differential diagnosis and/or concern for intellectual disability. They will require the use of standardized tools and consultation with specialists to make a diagnosis. In these cases, after complete review, the primary care clinician may be able to make a preliminary or provisional diagnosis and refer the child for support while the child awaits multidisciplinary evaluation to confirm the diagnosis. The discussion of findings and recommended therapies should occur as the primary care clinician and specialist collaborate to support the child and family.

Tier 3, more complicated cases requiring multidisciplinary evaluation: In the child with more complex and overlapping presentations or differential diagnoses, a referral for specialty assessment is made and simultaneous referrals for therapy are recommended for areas of delay.

Abbreviations: *DSM-5-TR, Diagnostic and Statistical Manual of Mental Disorders, Fifth Edition, Text Revision;* STAT, Screening Tool for Autism in Toddlers and Young Children.

Adapted with permission from Missouri Autism Guidelines Initiative. *Autism Spectrum Disorders: Missouri Best Practice Guidelines for Screening, Diagnosis, and Assessment; a 2010 Consensus Publication.* The Thompson Foundation for Autism and the Division of Developmental Disabilities, Missouri Department of Mental Health; 2010. Accessed February 27, 2026. https://dmh.mo.gov/media/pdf/autism-guidelines.

The level I screeners available for use are reviewed in Chapter 5, Autism Screening in Primary Care. The Childhood Autism Spectrum Test (CAST) is a free screening questionnaire used for children aged 4 to 11 years. The Social Responsiveness Scale, Second Edition (SRS-2), is used for ages 2.5 years to adulthood, and the Autism Spectrum Rating Scales (ASRS) are used for ages 2 to 18 years. The latter 2 screening tools are proprietary and incur fees. Each one has separate forms and scoring for teachers and parents. They each provide subscale ratings for specific developmental domains that can be useful in developing care goals. Both tools are available as paper questionnaires or can be completed online. The request for questionnaire completion can be emailed to the responder, and scoring is completed online and available to the clinician for minimal fees. Refer to **Table 5.1**, Autism Screening Tools, for descriptions and references.

Many primary care clinicians are now using a level II screener for children who are being evaluated for autism after an increased likelihood has been identified. The STAT can be easily performed in a primary care setting. It requires a specific set of toys, as well as standardized administration of each of the 12 items of the test. It has strong predictive value down to 16 months of age but requires 6 months of monthly or bimonthly training and supervision to reach fidelity. The time required to complete this assessment tool is a service that allows the clinician to more comfortably make a diagnosis and provide documentation to satisfy payment for services. A discussion of billing codes used for primary care screening and assessment is included in Chapter 4, The Pragmatics of the Pediatric Visit.

The RITA-T is another level II screener that has been validated in toddlers aged 18 to 36 months. Online training is available through centers such as Boston Children's Hospital and the Kennedy Krieger Institute. The RITA-T is an interactive and observational measure that can differentiate between a child on the autism spectrum and one with other developmental conditions. The training requires approximately 3 hours, and the exam requires 10 to 20 minutes of office time.

The CARS-2 is another quantitative measure used to codify and quantify clinical observations of a child. It is validated for age 2 years to adulthood and takes 10 minutes of administration after the history has been collected. It is meant to be administered by a clinician with autism experience, and a brief training in the use of the tool is required. The ratings are to be completed after the child is observed in an informal office interaction.

Additionally, there is an artificial intelligence–based US Food and Drug Administration–approved technology to allow for remote diagnosis of autism. This is the Canvas Dx technology produced by Cognoa. This technology requires input from a clinician, a detailed history from the family, and the analysis of home video clips to make a diagnosis in children aged 18 months to 6 years. This tool demonstrated a 94% positive predictive value with a 95% negative predictive value compared with in-person diagnostic evaluations.

Documenting Diagnostic Features in the Electronic Health Record

It is necessary to document what screening tools have been used and to document the specific diagnostic features that support the autism diagnosis. The observations consistent with the diagnosis should be specific to the *DSM-5-TR* diagnostic features. This correlation is easily accomplished by incorporating a saved list of *DSM* criteria into the EHR that can then be used in visit notes (refer to Appendix D, Diagnostic Criteria for Electronic Health Record Documentation). Alternatively, the completion of a checklist that can be scanned into the record can be used to document the *DSM* diagnostic features. One such checklist, provided by the team at Vanderbilt University, is referenced in Appendix E, Diagnostic Criteria Checklist With Developmental Anchors.

The Multidisciplinary Diagnostic Evaluation

When clinical suspicion for autism is present and the pediatric primary care clinician feels unable to make a definitive diagnosis, a child is referred for specialty evaluation by a developmental specialist or team with autism expertise. Coincident with the referral for evaluation, the child is referred for EI services. It is helpful for primary care clinicians to educate the family about what to expect at such an evaluation and then to meet with the family after the evaluation to review the findings of the team and the care plan. It is additionally possible that some of the components of the diagnostic evaluation will be completed by a variety of specialists and gathered by the primary care clinician to determine an autism diagnosis. The components of the evaluation are listed in **Box 6.2**.

BOX 6.2 Components of an Autism Evaluation

1. History: Elicitation of family, behavioral health, perinatal, and developmental histories; review of autism-specific concerns and any coexisting conditions. Refer to Appendix C, Sample Intake Questionnaire, for a detailed example of an intake questionnaire.
2. Review of concern identified by other caregivers, child care providers, or teachers: This may include the use of standardized questionnaires, such as the SRS-2, SCQ, or ASRS.
3. Developmental evaluation including a review of language, motor, cognitive, and adaptive behaviors.
4. Hearing evaluation: Formalized behavioral audiological examination with an audiologist.
5. Physical examination including growth parameters (with head circumference), skin examination, neurological examination, and examination for possible dysmorphic features.
6. Autism assessment and play observation: ADOS-2, level II screener (the STAT or the RITA-T), or CARS-2.
7. Assessment of family supports and social drivers of health: Screening for housing and food security, financial stability, environmental context, family mental health, and exposures to potential trauma.
8. Sharing of feedback and a discussion of a care plan that is both culturally and linguistically accessible to the family.
9. Educational materials and community resources provided to the family.

Abbreviations: ADOS-2, Autism Diagnostic Observation Schedule, Second Edition; ASRS, Autism Spectrum Rating Scales; CARS-2, Childhood Autism Rating Scale, Second Edition; RITA-T, Rapid Interactive Screening Test for Autism in Toddlers; SCQ, Social Communication Questionnaire; SRS-2, Social Responsiveness Scale, Second Edition; STAT, Screening Tool for Autism in Toddlers and Young Children.

The team involved in evaluation for autism may consist of any combination of the following professionals:

- Speech pathologist
- Developmental pediatrician
- Neurologist
- Psychologist
- Psychiatrist
- Early childhood specialist
- Occupational therapist

The evaluation of a child for possible autism requires expertise with this population as well as thorough training in child development. These specialists have the expertise needed to obtain a thorough history from multiple observers and interact with and observe the child in unstructured play and to perform a formal diagnostic assessment. It is important to understand that the clinical presentation of autism may be complicated by the presence of overlapping behavioral health issues such as anxiety, a communication disorder, attention-deficit/hyperactivity disorder, an underlying medical entity, ID, or issues related to experienced trauma and/or other social drivers of health. Experienced trauma and significant familial stress may cause a child to exhibit dysregulated symptoms that appear similar to or add complexity to the concerns of autism. In some cases, an autistic-like presentation may be secondary to a different primary clinical entity, such as genetic causes of ID. It is children with more complexity who benefit from the expertise of autism specialists.

It can be difficult to successfully engage children on the autism spectrum in an assessment, and it can be challenging to elicit their optimal level of performance. Skilled diagnosticians are familiar with these issues and have the knowledge to gather information from many sources, the practice to take careful histories, and the skills to bring out the highest performance in children while observing for coexisting medical diagnoses. Such diagnosticians can use a variety of assessment tools that rely on different skill sets and areas of strength in the child. In the case of autism, many children have language difficulties, making assessment and determination of cognition more challenging. The reliance on language-based assessment tools and the determination of verbal cognition can provide falsely depressed cognitive scores. Optimally, the diagnostician will rely on tools that assess for and report on nonverbal cognitive abilities to obtain a more valid assessment of cognitive potential. Many clinicians assessing the autistic child will emphasize nonverbal cognition and either not report or de-emphasize verbal cognition.

Assessment protocols for autism diagnosis vary between different centers, as do the tools used. A thorough history must be reviewed, including family history and developmental, perinatal, medical, and psychosocial histories. Some centers have their own intake procedures or may rely on standardized questionnaires to collect this information. Academic centers tend to use the 2- to 3-hour Autism Diagnostic Interview, Revised (ADI-R). These standardized questionnaires collect information specific to autism and related entities and can be administered to child care providers, teachers, and parents.

The child will undergo assessments of developmental status or cognition, speech and language abilities, and play interaction, as well as a diagnostic assessment for autism. Many psychologists will use a variety of developmental tools that include assessments of skills related to autism in addition to the standard repertoire of autism assessment tools. The Autism Diagnostic Observation Schedule, Second Edition (ADOS-2); the CARS-2; and the STAT are the most commonly used direct assessment tools when evaluating a child for an autism diagnosis. The ADOS-2 requires intensive training and takes approximately 45 minutes to administer and score. There are different modules based on the language skill of the individual, and these modules can be administered to children 12 months of age to adulthood. The CARS-2 is another method for systematically observing a child during an unstructured interaction. It consists of a 15-point scale taken from history and observations. This tool can be extremely helpful in documentation for insurance purposes and can be either administered as a parent questionnaire or scored by using the clinician's observations during the course of a pediatric visit. This does not require a specific toolkit but does require a short training on administration and can be administered after observing the child in the office. The STAT (reviewed earlier in this chapter, in the Potential Role of the Pediatric Primary Care Clinician in Diagnosis section) is another tool, used when the child is 24 to 36 months of age.

As part of the multidisciplinary evaluation, the child will need to undergo an assessment of language, communication, and motor skills and some formal measure of cognition or developmental level. A formalized assessment of adaptive functioning is necessary to document the effects of a developmental condition such as autism on the child's everyday behavior. Many specialists in diagnostic centers and school systems will use the Vineland Adaptive Behavior Scales, Third Edition (Vineland-3), or the Adaptive Behavior Assessment System, Third Edition (ABAS-3), for this purpose.

Chapter 7, The Medical Evaluation of the Child Presumed or Confirmed to Be Autistic, discusses in detail the American Academy of Pediatrics recommendations for genetic testing and what is required of a medical evaluation for children who have received a diagnosis of autism. In summary, all children require a formal hearing evaluation and a physical examination to assess for contributing medical etiologies. Some autism specialists will perform genetic testing and other medical testing as indicated by the history or may leave the decision to pursue this testing to the pediatrician or a geneticist.

Formal evaluations conclude with a reporting of findings, specific diagnoses, and suggestions for care goals, including therapy. These recommendations may provide names of therapy centers or, in most cases, will provide general guidance to be followed by the family. Many autism specialists are not located within the family's community, so it is more relevant for the pediatric primary care clinician to have listings of local parent-run or nonprofit organizations to which they can refer families (refer to Appendix F, Parent Resources on Autism). It is important that the type and culture of the support align with the values of the family, and any language or logistical barriers should be reviewed with the family so their input is considered as recommendations are made.

The team's findings should include a comprehensive listing of areas of need requiring attention. The families will benefit from time reviewing these findings with the primary care clinician to understand and process these recommendations. The primary care clinician should be ready to assist with report interpretation and to provide resources in or near the family's community to help support the care plan. Parents will benefit from a brief discussion of the importance of evidence-based support and the options available in the region. Over time, parents should seek out local nonprofit and other organizations that provide parent support and education. Many of these organizations can assist with issues related to the special education system, the Medicaid waiver (qualifying for Medicaid based on developmental and/or medical need), and long-term planning for the family.

Barriers to Diagnosis

Despite the growing awareness of autism and services available for young children, there are persistent barriers to diagnosis and care that can exist for many families. As previously mentioned, many specialists have long wait lists, and families living in more remote settings may not have access to these professional services. Insurance coverage may be a real limitation, as not all evaluations are covered consistently by insurance providers. Some parents may not identify the same level of concern to alert a primary care clinician. Other parents report that the tools used to screen for and diagnose autism include questions or activities that are unfamiliar to their culture. The literature indicates that children with higher cognition are likely to be identified later due to their enhanced ability to meet developmental standards longer. Children of color are more likely to be diagnosed later, their parents are less likely to report feeling heard by the clinician, and the children may even be misdiagnosed with other behavioral health concerns before an autism diagnosis is made, raising concern about potential bias or challenges with access to diagnostic services. Children from higher socioeconomic groups whose parents express increased concern represent those who are more likely to be identified and referred earlier.

In addition, the validity of an autism diagnosis depends on a determination that the features of autism in the child create significant challenges. This determination can be limited by the child's lack of experiences in group settings outside the home. Early intervention childhood educators or therapists are valuable resources for this type of feedback. It can be helpful for the clinician to obtain the progress notes of these professionals or, ideally, to communicate with them about their observations and priorities.

Young children may not yet be identified by child care centers as exhibiting concerning developmental features. If the child's behavior is not disruptive to others and/or the child is able to entertain themselves, a child care provider may not raise concerns. Caregivers may appreciate the cognitive skill sets of a toddler who has learned to identify letters and early phonics and may therefore not appreciate how the nature of the child's ritualistic interest in these early academic skills may create challenges. Not all child care providers will have specific expectations or requirements of the child or express concern about subtle difficulties in social interaction and play. Further, at the earliest ages when autism can be diagnosed, the expectation for building friendships is limited. It can be challenging to meet the necessary criterion of struggling to engage with peers and establish friendships. That observation can require a sophisticated knowledge of early development to recognize subtler degrees of difficulty.

When a primary care clinician suspects that a child may be on the spectrum, it is helpful for them to ask questions related to the specific features of autism or administer questionnaires to the adults who care for the child in different settings. An observation of the child in a preschool or child care setting can be very helpful in understanding the child's level of functioning. Gathering the perspective of other adults in the child's life (relatives, teachers, and parents) can be helpful as well. If the child is firstborn and the parents do not have a standard for what is expected during typical development, it is particularly important to gather other adults' perspectives on the child's development.

Although most children identified as having an increased likelihood of autism are ultimately referred for specialty evaluation, the pediatric primary care clinician plays a critical role in the diagnostic process. As illustrated in the case vignette at the beginning of this chapter, the primary care clinician is often the first to hear parents' concerns and to identify the likelihood of autism through universal or targeted screening. When clinicians create opportunities for in-person encounters, parents frequently share additional observations and concerns. Ongoing support from the pediatric primary care clinician remains essential both before and after specialty evaluation, as families navigate parent support groups, educational resources, insurance reimbursement, and the wide range of community-based educational and therapeutic services.

CASE VIGNETTE: CONCLUSION

As their conversation with the primary care clinician continues, Jonah's parents begin to share more about their own concerns. In preschool, Jonah demonstrates little interest in his peers, does not join them in play, and will frequently hit peers who attempt to initiate play with him. He plays only with the block set and has difficulty transitioning away from this activity. He seems to have frequent tantrums when asked to transition or to follow a new or unexpected instruction. His parents are increasingly concerned about his behaviors and development. They are particularly concerned that he still uses words only when labeling his favorite objects, letters, and colors. When he wants something, he will use their hand to pull them to what he desires but does not communicate using gestures or words.

The primary care clinician shares that these features suggest a diagnosis of autism. The parents are tearful but express relief that someone has created an opportunity to talk about their concerns and the possibility of a cause for Jonah's behaviors and development. They had been blaming themselves for spending too much time at work and not finding ample social experiences for Jonah. The discussion now proceeds to a description of autism, the many strengths of those on the spectrum, and next steps.

The clinician writes a summary of Jonah's history and clinical findings and uses a templated copy of the *Diagnostic and Statistical Manual of Mental Disorders, Fifth Edition, Text Revision* (*DSM-5-TR*) criteria that had been created in the electronic health record (EHR) to make a provisional diagnosis of autism. The concerns identified from this visit lead the clinician to recommend a follow-up appointment for an assessment using standardized tools. A handout describing autism with educational resources is provided to the parents. They are referred for an early intervention (EI) assessment with Jonah's school district resources for special education services. Referrals for speech and occupational therapies are given to the family. For the clinician to have more time to observe the child, the parents are asked to return within a month to discuss the possibility of an autism-specific intervention, such as applied behavior therapy. At that next appointment, the primary care clinician plans to observe a play interaction and complete a Childhood Autism Rating Scale, Second Edition (CARS-2), assessment. She sends requests to the preschool teacher to complete a standardized autism questionnaire that will provide further data to contribute to the evaluation for autism.

Clinical Pearls

- The diagnosis of autism spectrum disorder is made when an individual presents with a behavioral profile that meets the *DSM-5-TR* criteria and is not attributed to global developmental delay or ID.
- Children on the autism spectrum present with a combination of difficulties in social engagement, reciprocity, and nonverbal communication in addition to the atypical, repetitive, restricted patterns of behavior and interests.
- The characteristics or traits of autism must create significant challenges for the child.
- The severity ratings are determined by the amount of support required for the child to successfully engage socially as well as the degree of difficulty resulting from the restricted and repetitive behaviors and interests.
- Many primary care clinicians are involved in autism diagnosis.
- In the tiered approach to diagnosis, the primary care clinician serves to triage children presenting with concern for autism. The primary care clinician is able, with training, to make valid diagnoses in children presenting with autism without a complexity of co-occurring conditions.
- A clinician's notes must contain thorough documentation of findings. There are many tools to assist with this.
- Specialists in autism diagnostic services have the expertise to obtain a thorough history from multiple observers, interact and observe the child in unstructured play, and perform a formal diagnostic assessment.
- The pediatric primary care clinician should refer the child for support while the family is awaiting diagnostic confirmation.
- The pediatric primary care clinician should review the diagnostic findings with the family and address questions and concerns the family has.

References

American Academy of Pediatrics. Autism diagnosis in primary care. Updated September 26, 2025. Accessed February 27, 2026. https://www.aap.org/en/patient-care/autism/autism-diagnosis-in-primary-care

American Academy of Pediatrics Committee on Children With Disabilities. The pediatrician's role in the diagnosis and management of autistic spectrum disorder in children. *Pediatrics.* 2001;107(5):1221–1226 PMID: 11331713 doi: 10.1542/peds.107.5.1221

Bellesheim KR, Kizzee RL, Curran A, Sohl K. ECHO Autism: integrating maintenance of certification with Extension for Community Healthcare Outcomes improves developmental screening. *J Dev Behav Pediatr.* 2020;41(6):420–427 PMID: 32735419 doi: 10.1097/DBP.0000000000000796

Brian JA, Zwaigenbaum L, Ip A. Standards of diagnostic assessment for autism spectrum disorder. *Paediatr Child Health.* 2019;24(7):444–451 PMID: 31660042 doi: 10.1093/pch/pxz117

Carbone PS, Campbell K, Wilkes J, et al. Primary care autism screening and later autism diagnosis. *Pediatrics.* 2020;146(2):e20192314 PMID: 32632024 doi: 10.1542/peds.2019-2314

Corona L, Hine J, Nicholson A, et al. *TELE-ASD-PEDS: A Telemedicine-based ASD Evaluation Tool for Toddlers and Young Children.* Vanderbilt University Medical Center; 2020. Accessed February 27, 2026. https://vkc.vumc.org/vkc/triad/tele-asd-peds

Di Renzo M, Guerriero V, Zavattini GC, Petrillo M, Racinaro L, Bianchi di Castelbianco F. Parental attunement, insightfulness, and acceptance of child diagnosis in parents of children with autism: clinical implications. *Front Psychol.* 2020;11:1849 PMID: 32849089 doi: 10.3389/fpsyg.2020.01849

Gabrielsen TP, Farley M, Speer L, Villalobos M, Baker CN, Miller J. Identifying autism in a brief observation. *Pediatrics.* 2015;135(2):e330–e338 PMID: 25583913 doi: 10.1542/peds.2014-1428

Guan X, Zwaigenbaum L, Sonnenberg LK. Building capacity for community pediatric autism diagnosis: a systemic review of physician training programs. *J Dev Behav Pediatr.* 2022;43(1):44–54 PMID: 34907998 doi: 10.1097/DBP.0000000000001042

Hyman SL, Levy SE, Myers SM, et al; American Academy of Pediatrics Council on Children With Disabilities and Section on Developmental and Behavioral Pediatrics. Identification, evaluation, and management of children with autism spectrum disorder. *Pediatrics.* 2020;145(1):e20193447 PMID: 31843864 doi: 10.1542/peds.2019-3447

Masi A, DeMayo MM, Glozier N, Guastella AJ. An overview of autism spectrum disorder, heterogeneity and treatment options. *Neurosci Bull.* 2017;33(2):183–193 PMID: 28213805 doi: 10.1007/s12264-017-0100-y

Mazurek MO, Curran A, Burnette C, Sohl K. ECHO Autism STAT: accelerating early access to autism diagnosis. *J Autism Dev Disord.* 2019;49(1):127–137 PMID: 30043354 doi: 10.1007/s10803-018-3696-5

Mazurek MO, Parker RA, Chan J, Kuhlthau K, Sohl K; ECHO Autism Collaborative. Effectiveness of the Extension for Community Health Outcomes model as applied to primary care for autism: a partial stepped-wedge randomized clinical trial. *JAMA Pediatr.* 2020;174(5):e196306 PMID: 32150229 doi: 10.1001/jamapediatrics.2019.6306

Missouri Autism Guidelines Initiative. *Autism Spectrum Disorders: Missouri Best Practice Guidelines for Screening, Diagnosis, and Assessment; A 2010 Consensus Publication.* The Thompson Foundation for Autism and the Division of Developmental Disabilities, Missouri Department of Mental Health; 2010. Accessed February 27, 2026. https://dmh.mo.gov/media/pdf/autism-guidelines

Myers L, Karp SM, Dietrich MS, Looman WS, Lutenbacher M. Family-centered care: how close do we get when talking to parents of children undergoing diagnosis for autism spectrum disorders? *J Autism Dev Disord.* 2021;51(9):3073–3084 PMID: 33140145 doi: 10.1007/s10803-020-04765-0

Myers SM. How likely is it that I could have another child with autism? Association for Science in Autism Treatment. Accessed February 27, 2026. https://asatonline.org/research-treatment/clinical-corner/recurrence-of-autism-in-families

National Library of Medicine. Autism spectrum disorder. MedlinePlus. Updated October 21, 2021. Accessed February 27, 2026. https://medlineplus.gov/genetics/condition/autism-spectrum-disorder/#causes

Pearson JN, Meadan H, Malone KM, Martin BM. Parent and professional experiences supporting African-American children with autism. *J Racial Ethn Health Disparities.* 2020;7(2):305–315 PMID: 31758417 doi: 10.1007/s40615-019-00659-9

Pierce K, Glatt SJ, Liptak GS, McIntyre LL. The power and promise of identifying autism early: insights from the search for clinical and biological markers. *Ann Clin Psychiatry.* 2009;21(3):132–147 PMID: 19758535

Richards M, Mossey J, Robins DL. Parents' concerns as they relate to their child's development and later diagnosis of autism spectrum disorder. *J Dev Behav Pediatr.* 2016;37(7):532–540 PMID: 27541581 doi: 10.1097/DBP.0000000000000339

Schieltz KM, Brown R, Nanclares-Nogués V, et al. Evaluating autism diagnosis agreement between primary care physicians/practitioners and experts through ECHO Autism STAT. *Res Autism Spectr Disord.* 2023;109:102276 doi: 10.1016/j.rasd.2023.102276

Sohl K, Levinstein L, James A, et al. ECHO (Extension for Community Healthcare Outcomes) Autism STAT: a diagnostic accuracy study of community-based primary care diagnosis of autism spectrum disorder. *J Dev Behav Pediatr.* 2023;44(3):e177–e184 PMID: 36978232 doi: 10.1097/DBP.0000000000001172

Visser JC, Rommelse NN, Lappenschaar M, Servatius-Oosterling IJ, Greven CU, Buitelaar JK. Variation in the early trajectories of autism symptoms is related to the development of language, cognition, and behavior problems. 2017;56(8):659–668 PMID: 28735695 doi: 10.1016/j.jaac.2017.05.022

Weitlauf AS, Miceli A, Vehorn A, et al. Screening, diagnosis, and intervention for autism: experiences of Black and multiracial families seeking care. *J Autism Dev Disord.* 2024;54(3):931–942 PMID: 36626007 doi: 10.1007/s10803-022-05861-z

CHAPTER

7

The Medical Evaluation of the Child Presumed or Confirmed to Be Autistic

CASE VIGNETTE

A family new to the practice brings their son, Mateo, to the office for his 3-year health supervision visit. During his time in the office, Mateo is very active, does not use any words or gestures, and pulls his parent's hand to get what he wants (eg, leaving the room, grabbing for the door). His parent reports that he does not speak any words yet and rocks repeatedly. He becomes upset easily and has taken to biting his wrist when he is denied a request. On examination, Mateo has an elongated face, somewhat enlarged ears, and low muscle tone. He does not make eye contact with the clinician or the parent and tends to chew on his wrist as he becomes agitated. There is immediate concern for possible autism given delays in his communication and social engagement as well as atypical repetitive features. Additionally, his physical examination has revealed dysmorphic features and suggested a medical cause for his atypical developmental presentation.

On further history, Mateo's mother reports that she has an adult brother who attended special education classes as a child and continues to live with their parents. He is unemployed and often exhibits behaviors that others find very disruptive. She additionally reports that she has a sister with a history of infertility and a relative in whom gait and balance difficulties developed later in life.

The clinician suspects that Mateo has fragile X syndrome and, after partnering with and asking permission from the parent, orders fragile x syndrome testing and refers Mateo to a geneticist or fragile x syndrome specialist for comprehensive developmental testing and guidance. In the interim, the clinician refers Mateo for early intervention services, private speech therapy, and a Medicaid waiver application. The Medicaid waiver program is a state-sponsored program by which a child with developmental disabilities undergoes a review of eligibility by the state to receive Medicaid coverage or support for

Continued on next page

home care (refer to Chapter 15, Long-Term Goals and Transition Planning: It Takes a Village). The clinician provides the parent with handouts that offer information to support play and communication, and a follow-up appointment is scheduled to review Mateo's progress and test results. The clinician explains that if the first set of genetic tests do not identify a cause for Mateo's delays, Mateo will need to undergo more comprehensive testing once the family meets with a geneticist.

Assessment of the child with a new or likely autism diagnosis should include a comprehensive review of their medical and developmental history and family history as well as a physical examination. The process of assessing for medical causes and co-occurring conditions seen in those on the autism spectrum is exemplified in the case vignette. The recommendations for the medical evaluation are well articulated in the American Academy of Pediatrics 2020 clinical report "Identification, Evaluation, and Management of Children With Autism Spectrum Disorder." This chapter discusses similar recommendations while providing additional tools for the clinician who engages in such an evaluation.

The autism diagnosis will likely be made by a team of specialists that may or may not include a medical professional. It is important that the pediatric clinician assess the need for further medical testing as indicated by findings from the history and the physical examination. There is a high co-occurrence of medical and behavioral health conditions associated with autism. These conditions and their treatments add additional medical risk and are a part of the assessment for medical testing. For a complete discussion of the conditions co-occurring with autism, refer to Chapters 10, Diagnosing and Managing Co-Occurring Conditions; 11, Gastrointestinal Symptoms and Feeding Challenges; and 12, Insomnia: Identification and Interventions.

Children on the spectrum who are being followed over their lifespan by their primary care clinician will require careful surveillance for the most frequently associated conditions. The occurrence of these conditions is summarized in **Table 7.1**. Note that the prevalence of these conditions varies depending on the source of the report and the type of population. Ranges are offered in **Table 7.1**.

Associated Risk Factors

The clinician must thoroughly examine the family's medical history, including any relevant illnesses, parental age, and fertility and pregnancy history (including exposures to substances such as tobacco), alongside a comprehensive perinatal record. These data are crucial for uncovering potential epigenetic and genetic factors that could predispose the child undergoing assessment and their siblings to autism and potentially linked medical conditions. (Refer to Appendix C, Sample Intake Questionnaire.)

Table 7.1. Medical Conditions Co-Occurring in Children on the Autism Spectrum

Condition	Prevalence Among Autistic Children, %
Motor dysfunctions	79
Gastrointestinal symptoms	Up to 70
Epilepsy	Up to 30
Intellectual disability	39.6 (IQ: ≤70), 24.2 borderline (IQ: 71–85)[a]
Sleep disorders	50–80
ADHD	50–80
Behavioral health and related: anxiety, depression, mood disorder, ADHD, tic disorders	Up to 70
Pica	Up to 25

Abbreviations: ADHD, attention-deficit/hyperactivity disorder; IQ, intelligence quotient.

[a] Shaw KA, Williams S, Patrick ME, et al. Prevalence and early identification of autism spectrum disorder among children aged 4 and 8 years—Autism and Developmental Disabilities Monitoring Network, 16 sites, United States, 2022. *MMWR Surveill Summ.* 2025;74(2):1–22.

Family History

Because genetic risk factors overlap for many neurodevelopmental disorders, a thorough family history should be elicited when a child is undergoing an autism diagnostic assessment or has recently received a diagnosis. The pediatric clinician should consider collecting this information when the formal autism evaluation is delayed by long wait times. The existence of related disorders in a family contributes to the child's individual likelihood of autism and associated medical conditions. The family history should include extended family members who received special education services or had delays in skills of independence as an adult. These individuals may have undiagnosed autism or other associated developmental conditions that are relevant to the genetic risk factors for the index child. Families will benefit from reviewing their history in more detail to collect an accurate family tree.

Specific review of the family history for the following conditions and disorders is recommended to determine contributing risk and possible co-occurrence in the child:

- Behavioral health and related conditions: depression, anxiety, bipolar disorders, schizophrenia, attention-deficit/hyperactivity disorder (ADHD), tic disorders
- Fragile X syndrome and associated conditions: ataxia, infertility, primary ovarian insufficiency
- Intellectual disability (ID)
- Learning challenges: special education services, support in skills of independence from family members or not able to sustain work
- Seizure

Assessing existing support systems, mental health status, and exposure to trauma and abuse, as well as housing and food security, is a necessary part of every pediatric encounter but is especially pertinent when a child has additional health needs. Families with autistic children often face heightened stress levels, regardless of preexisting stressors. The need to navigate the complexity of therapies and the child's education, financial strain from increased costs associated with the child's care, caregiver burnout, familial strain, and the need for constant vigilance in the care for the child all contribute to the increased stress experienced by the family. Providing referrals to local organizations offering support and education should be standard practice for clinicians caring for families with autistic children.

A comprehensive review of both medical and developmental history, along with consideration of social drivers of health, is pertinent not only for assessing medical risks but also for devising a comprehensive care plan.

Medical History

A review of medical history as well as a review of systems is required to clarify the medical needs of a child under consideration for or having already received a diagnosis of autism. The medical history should specifically include gastrointestinal (GI) symptoms (pain, irregular/inconsistent/painful stooling patterns, pica, gastroesophageal reflux disease symptoms, vomiting, and rejecting or spitting out of food), sleep history, seizure history, feeding history, and developmental regression. Developing an understanding of any presenting behavioral challenges will both identify areas of support needed and include an evaluation to better understand the source or function of the behaviors. In some situations, behavioral challenges may be a manifestation of the pain or discomfort associated with an underlying medical condition co-occurring in the autistic child (further discussed in Chapters 9, Autism and Behavioral Challenges: Why They Occur and How to Approach Them; 10, Diagnosing and Managing Co-Occurring Conditions; 11, Gastrointestinal Symptoms and Feeding Challenges; and 12, Insomnia: Identification and Interventions).

The autistic child is at risk for neurological challenges, but not every child requires a referral to a neurologist. In children on the autism spectrum, any type of seizure disorder may develop. The seizure risk is biphasic, peaking in the preschool years and then peaking again in adolescence. Subtle presentations such as a sleep disorder or developmental regression should be investigated when they occur in addition to the presence of persistent staring or tonic-clonic movement. To aid in this evaluation, clinicians can ask the family to share home videos of the child engaging in behaviors thought to represent a seizure. It can be helpful to know if the behaviors are voluntary and can be interrupted by making a loud sound or by firmly placing a hand onto the child. This will help determine the true risk for seizure in a population that is likely to display many atypical movements and behaviors.

Children on the spectrum may present with tics that are to be distinguished from stereotypical behaviors. Tics are sudden, involuntary movements or vocalizations that may be preceded by a premonitory urgency. Stereotypies, on the other hand, are repetitive movements that may be related to stress, self-soothing, or sensory experiences and are part of the defining criteria for autism. The other neurological manifestations of autism that may improve with occupational or speech therapy are motor planning difficulties, verbal apraxia (speech sound disorder), and coordination challenges despite having reached motor milestones.

There is some concern for an increased tendency toward autoimmune disorders and allergies in individuals on the spectrum. The same level of surveillance is needed as with any child, while keeping in mind that children with communication disorders struggle to alert others to their symptoms. It may therefore be necessary to specifically ask about associations of symptoms with seasons or specific exposures to further determine causation. Allergic disease, including that of the skin, can lead to increased discomfort and irritability and thereby contribute to the phenotypic presentation.

The Physical Examination

The physical examination of the autistic child can be extremely challenging for the child and may require repeated visits to complete. In addition to the physical examination that is typically performed, it is essential that growth parameters, including head circumference, are monitored along with body mass index (BMI). This information can be helpful in further identifying genetic risk factors or associated conditions such as eating challenges or adverse effects of medication.

A general neurological assessment is an essential component in the examination of the autistic child. It should include examining the child's fine and gross motor skills in addition to assessing muscle tone, symmetry, strength, and reflexes and looking for a Gowers sign. An observation for possible dysmorphic features can help determine whether a genetic referral is indicated. A skin examination should evaluate for café au lait spots, axillary freckling, ash leaf spots, or neurofibromas as indicators of possible associated neurocutaneous syndromes. Refer to **Table 7.2** for features suggestive of a genetic syndrome or disorder in those on the autism spectrum.

The neurological evaluation can be challenging for any child, but for a child on the spectrum, it may be helpful to observe how the child's sensory vulnerabilities contribute to their anxiety during an assessment and adapt the assessment so the child feels more comfortable. Allowing the child to engage in a preferred type of play can be beneficial, as can working elements of the examination into playful interactions with the child. This is reviewed in more detail in Chapter 4, The Pragmatics of the Pediatric Visit, but ensuring that the child is prepared for each step, slowing the pace of the examination, and allowing the child some control

Table 7.2. Genetic Syndromes and Disorders Associated With Autism

Syndrome or Disorder	Genetic Variant/ Deletion	Clinical Features	Inheritance	Prevalence
Angelman syndrome	*UBE3A* deletions; bands 15q11–13	• Hypotonia • Little speech • Poor sleep • Seizures • Feeding challenges over the lifespan • Slow development • ID • Various physical features	Maternal inheritance	Rare
Duchenne muscular dystrophy	Band Xp21.2 deletion	• Hypotonia • Proximal muscular weakness	X-linked dominant	1/3,600 live male births; autism prevalence: 3.1%–20.7%[a]
Fragile X syndrome	Variation in *FMR1* gene on X chromosome	• Developmental delay • ID • Physical features: long jaw, high forehead, large ears, hyperextensible joints, postpubertal testicular enlargement	X-linked dominant	1/7,000 males and 1/11,000 females; 1%–6% of all people on the autism spectrum
Landau-Kleffner syndrome	Rare cause of epilepsy	• Developmental regression, acquired aphasia, auditory verbal agnosia	Unknown	Rare
Neurofibromatosis	*NF1* or *NF2* gene variation	• Café au lait spots • Axillary freckling • Lisch nodules • Neurofibromas • Learning disabilities • Attention-deficit/ hyperactivity disorder • Macrocephaly • Short stature	Autosomal dominant	1/3,000 live births
Phelan-McDermid syndrome	Band 22q13.3 deletion	• Hypotonia • Developmental delay/regression • ID • Delayed language skills	Unknown	1/30,000 live births; 1% of all people on the autism spectrum

Table 7.2 (*continued*)

Syndrome or Disorder	Genetic Variant/ Deletion	Clinical Features	Inheritance	Prevalence
PTEN mutations	*PTEN* gene variation	• Hamartoma tumor syndrome • Macrocephaly • ID	Autosomal dominant	Rare; 10%–20% of those on the spectrum with macrocephaly
Rett syndrome	*MECP2* variation	• Microcephaly • Seizures • Postnatal onset • Ataxia • Tremor • Spasticity • Neurodegenerative changes/regression	X-linked dominant	1/8,500 females
Smith-Magenis syndrome	Band 17p11.2 de novo deletion	• Broad face • Prominent lower jaw • Full cheeks • Midface flattening • ID • Delayed language • Profound sleep disturbances • Behavioral challenges	Unknown	Rare; most diagnosed individuals are autistic.
Trisomy 21/Down syndrome	Extra chromosome 21	• Hypotonia • ID • Flat facies • Single palmar crease • Various physical features	Nondisjunction	1/700 live births; 16%–18% meet criteria for autism.
Prader-Willi syndrome	*UBE3A* deletions; bands 15q11–13	• Muscular weakness • Feeding challenges in infancy • Slow development • ID • Obesity • Narrow forehead • Small hands and feet • Short stature	Paternal inheritance; de novo alteration	1/15,000 live births
Tuberous sclerosis complex	*TSC1* or *TSC2* variation	• Benign hamartomas • Developmental delay • Behavioral challenges • Ash leaf spots • Facial angiofibromas • Seizures • Shagreen patch • Periungual fibroma • Cardiac rhabdomyoma	Autosomal dominant	1/5,800 live births

Continued on next page

Table 7.2 *(continued)*

Syndrome or Disorder	Genetic Variant/ Deletion	Clinical Features	Inheritance	Prevalence
Velocardiofacial/ DiGeorge syndrome	Band 22q11.2 deletion	• Developmental delay • Congenital heart defect • Immunodeficiency • Small, low-set ears • Small palpebral fissures • Hooded eyes • Long face • Bulbous nose • Growth failure • Hypotonia • Immunodeficiency • Hypocalcemia coupled with cleft lip/palate	Autosomal dominant	Rare
Williams syndrome	Band 7q11.23 deletion	• Mild growth restriction • Low IQ • Anxiety • Loquacious behavior • Hoarse voice • Hyperverbal • Hypersensitivity to sound • Periorbital fullness • Anteverted nares • Long philtrum • Prominent lips • Supravalvular aortic stenosis • Renal artery stenosis • Partial anodontia	Autosomal dominant	1/7,500–10,000 live births

Abbreviations: ID, intellectual disability; IQ, intelligence quotient.

[a] Parisi L, Di Filippo T, Glorioso P, La Grutta S, Epifanio MS, Roccella M. Autism spectrum disorders in children affected by Duchenne muscular dystrophy. *Minerva Pediatr.* 2018;70(3):233–239.

over the interaction can also be helpful. The parent is likely to have suggestions that may result in the child feeling more comfortable. If the child is interested in the clinician's reflex hammer, for example, the clinician may allow the child to handle and to experiment safely with a second hammer. It may be beneficial to demonstrate specific and more intrusive parts of the physical examination (eg, of the ear or heart examination) on a parent or doll or to allow the child to engage with a preferred toy or a screen to distract them from the examination. Breaking the examination into segments with rests between steps may minimize the stress the child experiences. In all cases, prioritizing the aspects of the examination that are essential to the visit and then collecting other aspects by observations can make the visit more easily tolerated by the child. A clinician may observe, for instance, how the child uses their body to step up, jump, and perform fine motor activities in order to assess symmetry, strength, and gross and fine motor skills.

Toe walking is particularly common in children on the spectrum, and an examination of range of motion at the ankle to evaluate for possible tight heel cords is important to determine whether physical therapy and/or orthotic devices would be beneficial. Other causes of toe walking, such as cerebral palsy and spasticity, should be considered as well.

Medical Testing

All children receiving or being considered for a diagnosis of autism should undergo a formal audiological evaluation. If the child cannot participate in a behavioral audiological examination, referral for brainstem auditory evoked response testing is recommended. Additionally, visual screening should be conducted in the office, and children with visual concerns should be referred to an ophthalmologist specializing in young children with developmental challenges.

Maintaining dental health is crucial. Consistent vigilance and regular dental hygiene visits are essential to prevent and detect issues early. Since individuals on the autism spectrum may not communicate pain until it becomes severe, proactive monitoring is particularly important.

The only other routine testing recommended for the autistic child is genetic testing. As reviewed in Chapter 2, Demographics, Etiology, and Clinical Presentation, chromosomal microarray analysis (CMA) was recommended as a first-tier assessment by the American College of Medical Genetics and Genomics in 2011 for all children who have received a diagnosis of autism. All boys on the spectrum should undergo testing for fragile X syndrome CGG repeat analysis. In girls, this testing is indicated only when there is specific concern for fragile X syndrome. In addition, children on the spectrum with macrocephaly should undergo testing for possible *PTEN* gene variation, and girls with psychomotor regression, microcephaly, and seizures in addition to autism should be tested for a variation in the *MECP2* gene. Chromosomal microarray analysis is costly and should be accompanied by genetic counseling. It should therefore be accomplished by a referral to a geneticist. The genetics specialist is equipped to obtain insurance approval and appeal any insurance denials. Genetics referrals for all children on the spectrum are not practical. Access to a geneticist may be limited, or the family may not be interested in pursuing this type of evaluation. The alternative to such a referral is a buccal swab analysis performed in the office or home through a company that will first obtain preapproval from the insurance company, provide genetic counseling, and provide assurance that the family's financial responsibility will be kept to a minimum. Clinicians should work to ensure that if the family chooses not to have CMA testing performed, all male children will undergo testing for fragile X syndrome. This is relatively inexpensive and will likely be covered by most insurers.

Children with abnormal findings on neurological examination or history may be referred to a neurologist, especially if there is concern for a neurocutaneous syndrome, fetal alcohol spectrum disorder, muscular dystrophy, or a seizure disorder. Only children with focal neurological findings or abnormal electroencephalographic findings should undergo head imaging. Children with specific dysmorphic patterns may either be referred to a geneticist or be recommended for specific fluorescence in situ hybridization testing to rule out a specific syndrome (refer to **Table 7.2**). Other findings on the examination may determine types of testing, such as a Gowers sign prompting the clinician to obtain a creatine kinase level, skin findings indicating possible neurofibromatosis, or fetal alcohol spectrum disorder indicating the need for head imaging.

Children on the spectrum will need ongoing medical monitoring for various purposes. Of individuals on the spectrum, 27% to 80% are likely to receive at least one psychotherapeutic medication to address issues such as aggression, irritability, anxiety, depression, and ADHD-related symptoms. Those with behavioral health conditions may be prescribed more than one such medication. Those prescribed second-generation antipsychotics are at risk for metabolic syndrome and should be counseled about this risk. The clinician should also track the growth, BMI, blood pressure, and biannual glucose and lipid test results of any child taking a second-generation antipsychotic medication.

There is a growing understanding that individuals on the spectrum are more susceptible to obesity, inadequate nutrition, lack of physical activity, possible osteoporosis, and cardiovascular issues. Research into nutritional deficiencies reveals a range of observations. Individuals with selective eating patterns may have insufficient intake of key nutrients such as protein, iron, calcium, vitamin D, vitamin B_{12}, vitamin C, and/or fiber. Children with pica should be evaluated for possible iron and/or zinc deficiency and lead poisoning. It is important to consider the individual's history in determining which children should undergo nutritional screening.

Different forms of testing might be prompted by the presence of related conditions. Indications of concurrent conditions might manifest with nonspecific symptoms such as sleep disturbances, faltering growth, feeding challenges, developmental regression, or behavioral changes. A significant number of these cases may necessitate specialist assessment when such symptoms coincide with more distinct markers, such as food aversion, constipation, or weight loss. Typically, a lower threshold for referral and evaluation is taken for conditions such as celiac disease, gastroesophageal reflux disease, eosinophilic esophagitis, allergic or autoimmune disorders, or seizure conditions in those on the spectrum because of the lack of specific presentations.

Evaluations for possible metabolic etiologies in autism are performed rarely and are best managed by a specialist when one or more of the indicators listed in **Box 7.1** are present.

BOX 7.1 Indications for Metabolic Testing of Children on the Autism Spectrum

- Developmental regression
- Family history of metabolic disease
- Consanguinity
- Episodic deterioration, especially with illness or cyclic vomiting
- Enlarged organs
- Coarse facial features
- Movement disorders or ataxia
- Lack of newborn screening
- Acid-base or electrolyte imbalance

Clinical Pearls

- All children receiving or being considered for an autism diagnosis should undergo the following medical evaluations:
  - A careful review of medical, developmental, and family histories.
  - Developmental surveillance focusing on possible motor dysfunctions, epilepsy, global delay or ID, sleep disorders, GI symptoms and feeding challenges, and behavioral health concerns.
  - Universal screening of hearing, vision screening, and genetic testing (CMA and fragile X syndrome testing). Ensure that all children have regular dental examinations.
  - A careful review of possible adverse childhood events and familial stress, which is particularly important in the context of autism.
- All other medical testing is individually determined by findings from the history and a thorough physical examination.
- The pediatric primary care clinician is critical in this surveillance (Chapters 10, Diagnosing and Managing Co-Occurring Conditions; 11, Gastrointestinal Symptoms and Feeding Challenges; 12, Insomnia: Identification and Interventions; and 13, Review of Pharmacotherapy and Complementary Interventions, provide more guidance in this process).

References

Howe YJ, Palumbo ML, Neumeyer A. Medical evaluation of patients with autism spectrum disorder. In: McDougle C, ed. *Autism Spectrum Disorder.* Oxford University Press; 2015 doi: 10.1093/med/9780199349722.003.0005

Hyman SL, Levy SE, Myers SM, et al; American Academy of Pediatrics Council on Children With Disabilities and Section on Developmental and Behavioral Pediatrics. Identification, evaluation, and management of children with autism spectrum disorder. *Pediatrics.* 2020;145(1):e20193447 PMID: 31843864 doi: 10.1542/peds.2019-3447

Rylaarsdam L, Guemez-Gamboa A. Genetic causes and modifiers of autism spectrum disorder. *Front Cell Neurosci.* 2019;13:385 PMID: 31481879 doi: 10.3389/fncel.2019.00385

Shaw KA, Williams S, Patrick ME, et al. Prevalence and early identification of autism spectrum disorder among children aged 4 and 8 years—Autism and Developmental Disabilities Monitoring Network, 16 sites, United States, 2022. *MMWR Surveill Summ.* 2025;74(2):1–22 PMID: 40232988 doi: 10.15585/mmwr.ss7402a1

CHAPTER

8

Evidence-Based Supports and Services

CASE VIGNETTE

Rohan is a 4-year-old who received a diagnosis of autism around his second birthday. His parents bring him to the office for a visit in the fall to discuss his autism care plan. The pediatric primary care clinician has a copy of a thorough multidisciplinary assessment that the school performed as well as one of the developmental assessments that an autism care team administered the year prior.

Rohan has been attending a full-time autism-centered preschool at his local elementary school. His parents wonder if they should consider additional services at this time. They note that Rohan has many strengths but that his progress across all developmental domains has been limited. They express concern about his options for kindergarten. Rohan's parents bring his individualized education program (IEP) and progress reports, which document their concerns.

Rohan has a strong vocabulary and is an intelligent child. His assessments demonstrate age-appropriate cognitive abilities and strong language skills. They also demonstrate marked delays in language pragmatics and social engagement. In school, he shows little interest in his peers and has difficulty transitioning from his focused interests to lessons within the classroom. He gets very upset when asked to transition and when directed to perform nonpreferred tasks. Recently, his behavioral responses have heightened in such a way that he may throw objects, hit others, and run from the classroom when asked to perform a task he is not interested in. His teacher at school has concerns for the safety of other children, and when his behavior escalates, she is unable to engage him in a safe manner. To keep the classroom managed, she has him move to the hall with the teacher's aide. He is successful at avoiding demands and happily spends time in the hall with the teacher's aide. His parents acknowledge that they have similar struggles at home.

Understanding Options for Therapy

The governing principle in caring for children on the autism spectrum is that the therapy program must be tailored to the needs, expectations, and pragmatics of each child and family. Each child on the spectrum presents with their own constellation of strengths and challenges; therefore, referrals should be individualized, and each child should be cared for on the basis of their unique panel of developmental skills. This approach is highlighted by the maxim of professionals in the field: "If you have met one child on the spectrum, you have met one child on the spectrum." For the busy primary care clinician, the lack of a singular approach to therapy can be overwhelming, especially when a parent is seeking guidance. Despite how well articulated the published practice parameters are, the reality of providing therapy recommendations is complex and individually tailored to the needs of the child and family, their finances, and the pragmatics of the services available.

Families make choices based on their own beliefs and cultural practices, recommendations made to them, and the pragmatics of obtaining care. Some families may rely on publicly funded early intervention (EI) and special education services and do not have the resources or inclination to pursue outside private therapy. Some families may have a parent available who can obtain training to become an effective therapist and work with the child, while other parents choose to take their child to see a professional and rely on that individual to provide the services needed. No one approach works for all families, but some combination of parent involvement and reliance on autism-trained professionals is the general expectation.

There are guiding principles that can support the primary care clinician in providing optimal individualized care for children on the spectrum. The research demonstrates that an autism-specific manualized approach that is evidence based results in significant developmental progress compared to services that are regularly available in communities at public expense. Private therapies may be administered by autism specialists who use evidence-based approaches specific to autism or who may use the general interventions supportive of children with developmental delays. The therapy is provided most often in a one-on-one setting with the child. Parent involvement is variable, but preferably the parent receives regular updates about successes, amended goals, and training to continue the work at home. Publicly funded EI is performed by EI specialists in the home for the first 1 to 3 years (depending on the county). After this home-based programming, the child transfers into a preschool setting in which the curriculum may or may not be autism specific, teachers have variable levels of expertise, and the teacher to student ratio is variable. Special educators are trained to understand autism, its characteristics, and how to implement evidence-based approaches but rarely receive certification in these types of therapies. In a school-based program, the emphasis is on creating more inclusive learning environments, providing positive behavioral supports, creating sensory-supportive environments, and individualizing the teaching for each child. It is important that families understand the distinction between what is offered in the public school system and what is offered in a specialized autism therapy program. The bulk of families use some combination of publicly funded general developmental services and private therapy services during the preschool years and then tend to rely more heavily on services provided by schools during primary and secondary education. The role of the primary care clinician is to review a child's developmental progress, help families ensure that care goals are adequately comprehensive, and discuss the need for expansion of services when indicated. **Box 8.1** outlines the central principles and information that effectively guide the approach to autism therapy.

BOX 8.1 Core Principles of Autism Therapy

- **Therapy should aim to be comprehensive.**
- **The therapy is specific to autism and follows a curriculum that is evidence based.** (Refer to the Autism Therapies section later in this chapter.)
- **Service providers are expected to have specific autism training and expertise.**
- **All developmental domains will be targeted.** If possible, the intervention will target all developmental domains that are relevant or underdeveloped or lagging for a particular child. These may include social-emotional development, behavioral regulation, executive function skills, functional communication (as opposed to limiting teaching to vocabulary and academic skills), motor skills, adaptive skills, cognitive abilities, safety, and behavioral health.
- **A parent component is to be included.** Therapy is expected to include a parent training component during which providers meet regularly with parents to teach methods, elicit concerns, and monitor response to therapy. It has been demonstrated repeatedly that parent-led methods, in which parents have been trained, are equally effective and augmentative to professionally administered services.
- **Response to therapy will be assessed.** A care plan should contain a component for assessing progress and response to therapy. Schools will provide quarterly reports demonstrating progress toward therapeutic goals. Other private therapies have different methods of documenting progress and refining goals.
- **A system for daily communication is established.** Many educators and therapists will have a system for daily communication with the parents. Daily checklists of common behaviors and targeted skills provide easy ways for parents to receive feedback. Additionally, there should be opportunity for periodic review with parents and for tailoring of therapy after parent discussion.
- **Goals are relevant for the family.** The goals of therapy are flexible to allow for the prioritization of goals that are meaningful to and relevant for the family.
- **Private therapy organizations provide families with data about their practice.** Companies providing private therapy may be able to demonstrate a track record of retaining therapists and prioritizing consistency of the staff involved with each child.

Continued on next page

BOX 8.1 *(continued)*

- **Care is coordinated between therapy and school settings.** It is important for coordination of therapy goals and methods to occur across settings or services. A private therapist will ideally be willing to attend individualized education program meetings and meet with teachers to facilitate coordination of care between the therapy and school settings.
- **An emphasis on case management optimizes care.** An emphasis on case management is helpful for all children and families. Ideally, the pediatric primary care clinician along with specialists and the care team may serve collaboratively as case managers to monitor therapy, including its efficacy and fidelity, and communicate with the parents and other professionals on the team. The emphasis should be on the whole child and not just on specific skills. Case managers can ensure that the team periodically reviews therapy goals and methods.
- **Placement in the least restrictive environment is essential for inclusion.** The ultimate goal of intervention is to promote inclusion by placing the child into the *least restrictive environment,* with the aim of general education/mainstream placement if possible. Despite this lifetime goal, there may be times when a child will require intensive therapy in a special education setting, especially during the preschool years. There may be other children for whom a general education placement will not be possible because of the amount of support the child requires. Often the preschooler will require special education placement exclusively, while later primary and secondary schooling may consist of a combination of special and general education services. The child is likely to be placed into some combination of a general education environment and/or a smaller special education classroom. This balance is individually determined and varies depending on the services available in schools in each region. In addition to academics, many children on the spectrum benefit from autism-specific teaching focusing on communication, social engagement, and the skills of daily living.
- **Teaching life skills is a priority of intervention.** A priority should be placed on teaching life skills, such as maintaining hygiene, dressing, going to the store, using safe behavior, toileting, practicing self-regulation of emotional responses, managing difficulties with sensory processing, demonstrating appropriate social etiquette, and applying dating skills.
- **Teaching life skills is followed by teaching generalization of those skills.** Once skills are taught, there should be a system for teaching the generalization or spontaneous use of these skills in multiple settings. In other words, skills taught in a structured therapy session should then be taught within a variety of everyday settings, such as in social interactions, during eating and play, on the playground, and in the home.

Using Data to Guide Therapy

A comprehensive assessment of the autistic child serves to provide data that guide the choice of therapy goals. It is important that the parent obtain copies of these data to be shared and reviewed with the pediatric primary care clinician. The parent should also request a copy of the child's full IEP or individualized family service plan each year for review at health supervision visits. A comprehensive psychoeducational assessment should ideally be performed upon diagnosis and every 3 years thereafter unless there are specific areas that require interim evaluation. The primary care clinician can and should inform the parent that public school systems are required to provide these assessments or direct parents to private psychologists, advocates, and neuropsychologists who will perform the testing. It is helpful for the primary care clinician to review this information to obtain knowledge of the child's progress. This knowledge should inform intervention decisions and thoughts about the child's developmental trajectory.

Parents may seek guidance from the primary care clinician when there are concerns. Further, there may be times when a school system determines that an evaluation is unnecessary. Skipping such an evaluation should be discouraged, as this information is very informative and helps identify trends that better predict long-term potential.

These periodic psychological and educational assessments should ideally be composed of each of the following measures:

1. **A measure of the child's cognitive/developmental status:** This is viewed as the cognitive potential. Many individuals on the autism spectrum struggle to participate optimally in psychological assessments, so it may take an experienced practitioner with access to a variety of tools to successfully assess a child's cognitive potential. Individuals on the spectrum often struggle with verbal processing and abstract ideas, and as a result, nonverbal cognitive tests are better predictors of a child's cognitive potential. Often a practitioner will choose a test that is less reliant on verbal skills or report only the nonverbal cognitive performance. For a younger child, a developmental quotient (DQ) will be reported, and for an older child, when the results are believed to be more predictive of adult cognition, an intelligence quotient (IQ) is reported. It is helpful to have an assessment of the cognitive functioning of the autistic child, as there is often specific divergence (eg, language processing, verbal comprehension) that has significant effects and should be defined. In addition, it is important to distinguish children for whom a primary global developmental delay or an intellectual disability explains their presentation. Following are tests of cognition that may be used in assessment:
    - The Mullen Scales of Early Learning (MSEL): A tool used to assess language, motor, and perceptual abilities from birth to 68 months of age.
    - The Bayley Scales of Infant and Toddler Development, Third Edition (Bayley III): An assessment used to identify delays in cognitive, language, and/or motor development for ages 1 to 42 months.
    - The Wechsler Intelligence Scale for Children, Fifth Edition (WISC-V): A test that measures 5 cognitive domains to define intellectual ability in a child aged 6 to 12 years.

- The Differential Abilities Scales, Second Edition (DAS-II): A test designed to yield a broad index of intelligence by subtests that measure verbal ability, nonverbal reasoning, and spatial ability. These scales are often used for children who have delays in verbal abilities.
- The Leiter International Performance Scale, Third Edition (Leiter-3): A nonverbal test of intelligence and cognitive abilities based on problem-solving for ages 3 years and older.
- The Wechsler Preschool and Primary Scale of Intelligence, Fourth Edition (WPPSI-IV): An intelligence test for children aged 2.5 to 7 years 7 months. This test provides verbal and performance cognitive domain scores as well as a composite score.

2. **A measure of the child's functional level of achievement:** The gap between cognition and achievement identifies areas that require support. It is through this type of achievement testing that learning disabilities can be defined. Following are tests for this portion of the assessment:
   - The Kaufman Test of Educational Achievement, Third Edition (KTEA-3): A test used to evaluate academic skills in individuals aged 4 to 26 years.
   - The Woodcock-Johnson IV (WJ IV): A test used to assess cognitive abilities and 8 areas of academic functioning for ages 2 years through adulthood.
   - The Verbal Behavior Milestones Assessment and Placement Program (VB-MAPP): An assessment tool used for children on the spectrum to assess language and social skills.
3. **A measure of the child's skills of daily living (activities of daily living or adaptive behaviors):**
   - The Vineland Adaptive Behavior Scales, Third Edition (Vineland-3): Measures adaptive behavior by using a structured interview. These data can be used to support a diagnosis of autism and determine eligibility for special education and related programming.
   - The Adaptive Behavior Assessment System, Third Edition (ABAS-3): A standardized questionnaire for caregivers to assess complete adaptive skills. This tool is used from birth through adulthood.
4. **Responses from parent and teacher standardized questionnaires,** including additional information relevant to a child's profile such as areas of executive function, behavioral challenges, and characteristics or traits suggestive of attention-deficit/hyperactivity disorder (ADHD) or autism.
   - The Behavior Rating Inventory of Executive Function (BRIEF): A measure of executive function and self-regulation skills.
   - The Behavior Assessment System for Children, Third Edition (BASC-3): A set of rating scales to help professionals understand the behaviors and emotions that may be affecting a child's functioning.

- The Vanderbilt Assessment Scales (https://publications.aap.org/pediatriccare/resources/17510/Vanderbilt-Assessment-Scales; used for children aged 6–12 years) and the Conners, Third Edition (Conners 3; used for children and adolescents aged 6–18 years): Questionnaires administered to parents and teachers when a diagnosis of ADHD is being considered.
- The Autism Spectrum Rating Scales (ASRS) or the Social Responsiveness Scale, Second Edition (SRS-2): Teacher and parent scales for autism. Each has subscale ratings that may further identify areas that require support and document the effect of the child's autism within the context of the classroom.

5 **Speech and language assessment** should cover the following areas:

- Phonology: speech production, intelligibility
- Oral-motor function
- Receptive vocabulary
- Expressive vocabulary
- Semantics (vocabulary), grammar, morphology
- Language pragmatics: the use of language within a social context as exemplified by conversational skills, including turn taking, making requests, and responding
- Literacy skills: comprehension of text as well as creation of language to demonstrate knowledge
- Narrative skills: ability to tell a story

Typical tests used by speech pathologists may include the following ones:

- The Peabody Picture Vocabulary Test, Fifth Edition (PPVT-5): Measures receptive vocabulary for ages 2.5 years through adulthood.
- The Clinical Evaluation of Language Fundamentals, Fifth Edition (CELF-5): Measures core language and receptive and expressive vocabulary, as well as language structure and content, used for 5- to 22-year-olds.
- The Preschool Language Scales, Fifth Edition (PLS-5): A tool used to measure language from birth to 8 years of age. It assesses preverbal interaction in the youngest age range through literacy skills and provides scores for total language, comprehension, and expressive communication.
- The Test of Pragmatic Language, Second Edition (TOPL-2): Assesses social communication in context while evaluating listening skills, expression of feelings, making requests, and sustaining communication. This tool is used for students aged 6 to 19 years.

6. **Occupational and sensory processing assessment** to assess for fine motor skills, motor planning skills, visual motor skills, and the relevance of responses to sensory input.
7. **Narratives of observations:** Qualitative descriptions of a child's classroom behavior can be extremely informative. A professional from the child's educational team will observe and document the observations of a child during structured and unstructured classroom time. This description will focus on a child's behavioral responses to peers, demands made by the environment, academic functioning, emotional responses, and skills of independence.

Autism Therapies

There are many therapies that have been developed for and demonstrate efficacy in autism care. A comprehensive discussion of the most commonly available autism therapies is provided in the Autism Therapy Methods section later in this chapter. Recommendations for specific therapies are typically made based on the ease of obtaining these services, their affordability, their relevance for the child, and parent preferences. In many areas, ABA is the only autism-specific therapy that is covered by insurance and is readily available. Until recently, ABA was the primary approach, with adequate research data supporting its efficacy. More recent data show that several of the programs providing a combined behavioral and child-led style of therapy within a natural environment significantly strengthen language and communication over the long term. Further, concern has been identified about the efficacy data used to justify ABA therapy. A recent meta-analysis showed that many of the studies that supported ABA's efficacy may have been biased because they used parents or therapists who were invested in the outcome to assess response to therapy. Applied behavior analysis today should combine its use of natural environment teaching with structured teaching at the table that focuses on teaching specific skills.

The ABA approach uses a structured system to teach specific skills. Children cared for in this fashion often receive ABA services for more than 20 hours per week. Other methods, including the Early Start Denver Model; Joint Attention, Symbolic Play, Engagement and Regulation; and the Preschool Autism Communication Trial, are taught within the natural environment of the home or a child care setting, within the context of play and interaction. These natural process methods are less time consuming but have been demonstrated to be effective.

When families visit the pediatric primary care clinician to discuss therapeutic options for their child on the autism spectrum, they should be educated about the variety of supports and services available. The primary care clinician or a care navigator in the practice should become familiar with the recommendations from the research literature as well as the factors that determine which providers deliver care appropriate for each child. Taking into consideration insurance coverage, location, personal preferences, and what is known about the practice of each provider will help determine which type of care and which specific provider are recommended. Many families will perform their own research and rely on parent recommendations, insurance coverage, or logistical factors to make choices. The subjective response of the parent to a provider is valid. Some families will have strong preferences based on factors that are personal, such as the cultural orientation of the center, details of the physical plant, the experience they had while visiting the provider, or their subjective expectations for what they want for their child.

The research data of comparative analyses of autism therapy methods have many methodological weaknesses, and it is clear that better-designed prospective studies are needed to determine which elements of therapy are most effective. As a result, clinicians cannot make uniform and dogmatic recommendations for all children on the spectrum. The reality is that pragmatic considerations determine which referrals are made. Parents benefit from their pediatric clinician's guidance as they navigate the autism resources in their community. It is helpful for the pediatric practice to compile a list of providers in their community and to give families advice regarding the comparative advantages of the resources available.

Guidance for Choosing the Right Therapy for the Autistic Child

In most communities, the primary service available outside the public school system is ABA. This model of support for children on the autism spectrum has expanded significantly, driven both by increasing demand and by insurance providers' broad coverage of the model. Many centers now provide aspects of natural environment teaching with an opportunity for social interaction with peers that is similar to that in a school setting. In addition to intensive ABA therapies, often delivered in centers or in families' homes, many children receive speech and occupational therapies. Given this practical reality, an algorithm has been developed to provide a guide for clinicians supporting families as they navigate therapy options. This guide is based on data for therapy choices in addition to accumulated clinical experience. The algorithm is described in more detail in the following list.

There are many options for private therapy for autism. **Figure 8.1** provides one algorithm offering a model for selecting specific interventions. The pivotal choices illustrated are as follows:

1. **A thorough assessment of the child's developmental status serves as the foundation for therapeutic choices.** If the child has developmental delays with global impact, an intensive program, ideally with an intensive behavioral component, or an ABA program will most likely be recommended. If the child has age-appropriate skills or mild delays, the child should be screened for other significant barriers to success, including safety concerns (eg, elopement, pica,

climbing, running), mood concerns/irritability, aggression/disruptive behaviors, and possible emotional dysregulation. If these are present and felt to be of significance, a more intensive program is selected. Finally, an assessment of the child's needs in skills of independence and of the child's contributing family factors is included. Areas of identified need may determine which specific and integrated services a child may receive. More significant areas of need would suggest that more intensive and comprehensive therapy is indicated, typically placement into an ABA program of 20 to 40 hours per week. Parents should always be referred for support and education services.

2. **If the child has not progressed** in their existing therapeutic program after attempts to maximize therapies and further refine therapy goals, a discussion should take place with the family to consider more individualized and intensive programming, such as ABA.
3. **A discussion should take place regarding which type of ABA services are indicated** if a family has chosen this option. Would a child benefit most from a home- or center-based program? Some families prefer a home-based program that either augments or replaces services they receive through their child's public school. A parent must be present in the home for all home-based services. This type of ABA is provided by a registered behavior technician (RBT) who is remotely supervised by a master's-level Board Certified Behavior Analyst (BCBA). Parents who work, have several children, or manage a variety of competing demands may choose a center-based program. Center-based programs allow the child to receive full-time services with access to a variety of BCBAs in one building. Center-based programs provide more stability in the event of teacher attrition or illness. These programs often create a preschool-type experience for children who would benefit from a center-based setting, and this option can provide an opportunity for socialization, teach the generalization of skills in a variety of settings, and assist with school transitioning if/when the child moves to a less restrictive environment.
4. **All ABA therapy must include a regular parent training program.**
5. **Parents should receive regular communication** regarding the child's progress as well as everyday events.

Once the type of referral has been determined, discussion with the family about the use of criteria to select a quality provider is helpful. Pediatric clinicians working with families with a child on the spectrum will quickly learn that individual experiences with autism therapists vary widely. Since most families will work with ABA providers, a thorough discussion of how ABA centers can vary and what criteria can be used to choose an individual provider is beneficial. Some ABA providers offer only home-based services; some, only center-based. Some have comprehensive training programs for their technicians, while others hire only supervisory BCBAs who are experienced and have a track record for retention. Not

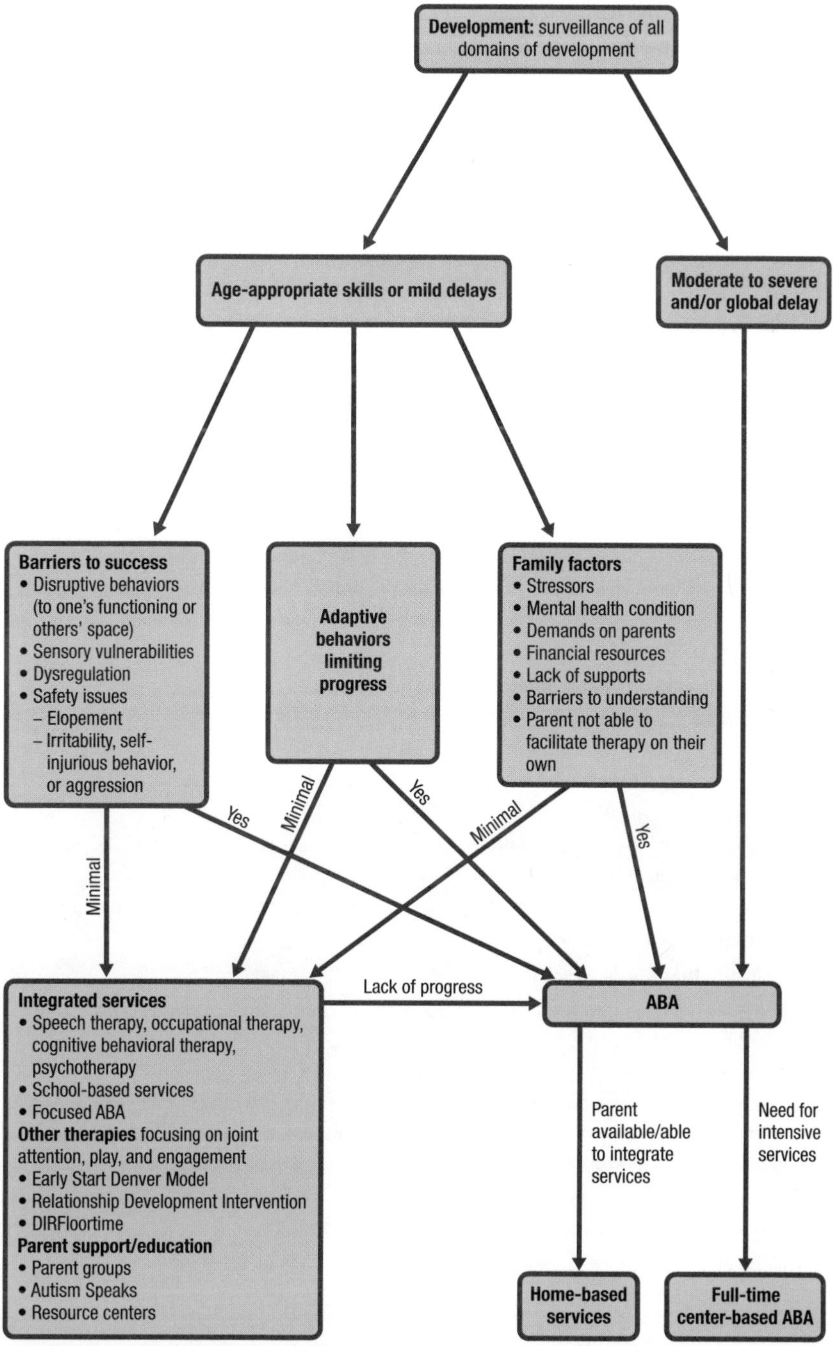

Figure 8.1. Practical Framework for Therapy Decisions

ABA indicates applied behavior analysis; DIRFloortime, Developmental, Individual-differences, and Relationship-based model.

all centers are equally family focused, with successful consideration of the inclusion of family needs and education. **Box 8.2** provides a list of criteria that can be used to select an ABA provider. These criteria can be extrapolated to the choice of any autism specialist.

BOX 8.2 Criteria Used to Select a Quality Applied Behavior Analysis Provider

1. Is the ABA provided within a center- or home-based program? Which is preferred for the child under consideration?
2. Is the ABA provider flexible with how many hours they can provide, or do they have a fixed approach? What are the minimum and maximum number of hours they will provide?
3. Does the ABA provider teach errorless learning? This method ensures that the child performs a task accurately before moving on.
4. How often will the family meet with the BCBA? What is the parent training component? Will the provider include treatment goals prioritized for and experienced by the family?
5. Will the child be assigned to a single therapist, or will the child work with a variety of therapists? If the child receives ABA therapy, the bulk of the therapy will be provided by a registered behavior technician. How is this person trained and supervised?
6. What has this center's therapist attrition rate been, and how do they handle absences when a therapist suddenly leaves or falls ill?
7. How experienced are the supervisory BCBAs? Have they received their degree? How many years of clinical experience do they have? How long have they worked for this particular provider?
8. Does the company have a contact person who is responsive and can assist with insurance approval, reimbursement, and payment plans?
9. How does the provider define treatment goals? Is the parent and/or other clinician allowed a role in defining goals?
10. Does the provider collaborate with the school, teachers, and therapists? Do they attend individualized education program meetings?
11. How long is the wait list? How long can the child receive services?
12. Can the provider supply references from other parents who have received services at their center?
13. Does the provider use principles from other methods such as the Early Start Denver Model and/or pivotal response therapy and have ample play-based teaching? Do the children enjoy attending? Is the program fun and developmentally appropriate? How much of the time is spent in tabletop (discrete trial) learning versus play? Are there opportunities to interact with other children?
14. Can parents tour the facility and/or speak with other parents?
15. Will the provider assist with transitions to new settings such as schools?

Abbreviations: ABA, applied behavior analysis; BCBA, Board Certified Behavior Analyst.

Autism Therapy Methods

Behavioral Approaches

Behavioral approaches incorporate the use of external reinforcers to encourage behaviors that are more desirable while reducing behaviors that are less desirable.

Applied behavior analysis (ABA): ABA uses methods from learning theory that rely on the assumption that behaviors develop when positive reinforcement is given. In ABA, a discrete stimulus is provided and a desired response is elicited and then reinforced by using extrinsic reinforcement (motivating snacks or access to toys or electronics). This behavioral approach is used to target a wide variety of developmental skills and behavioral challenges. Applied behavior analysis provides a systematic approach to assessment, teaching, and progress monitoring that is manualized, typically using the VB-MAPP tool. Therapy goals vary over time. When a goal is mastered, the child is taught to demonstrate generalization of the skill across different settings with progressively less support. Most ABA centers provide comprehensive programs of 20 to 40 hours of therapy per week. There are other programs that provide more problem-focused care by using behavioral services tailored to the individual's needs. Examples include specific behavioral concerns such as aggression, toileting issues, elopement or other safety issues, or challenges in skills of daily living. Children requiring this more focused ABA might be receiving other services elsewhere or not require a comprehensive ABA program.

When a child begins in an ABA program, a BCBA performs an assessment, assembles the therapy component of the care plan, and supervises the RBT who provides the therapy. The RBT receives training and ongoing supervision. Historically, these programs have been delivered in the home, but progressively, they are turning to a center-based model of care with an integrated parent component. There may be little flexibility about the number of hours each center will offer the family. Many states mandate insurance coverage for these services.

Discrete trial training (DTT): DTT is rarely used alone without the use of more natural environment teaching. It remains a part of ABA therapy and involves teaching specific skills in a systematic fashion to a child sitting at a table rather than integrating them into everyday learning, play, or interaction.

Picture Exchange Communication System (PECS): The PECS is a behaviorally reinforced method of teaching communication that is often integrated into a more comprehensive teaching program. The PECS is an effective method for teaching a nonspeaking child to use symbols for the purpose of communication. For instance, the child might reach for a picture of a specific food when making a request for that food. This may be a first step toward learning to communicate verbally.

Developmental Approaches

Developmental approaches to autism therapy are based on the notion that autism creates differences in social communication that may make it difficult to engage and interact with others. Delays in joint attention are thought to be responsible for the challenges in communication and learning. Therapy focuses on the synchrony of child-parent or therapist-child interactions through play. The expectation is that strengthening of joint attention will result in increased opportunities for learning.

DIRFloortime, also known as Floortime (from the Developmental, Individual-differences, and Relationship-based model): This model focuses on teaching engagement skills, play, and symbolic thinking embedded within play and social interaction. Learning occurs during child-led engagement when the provider modifies their level of affect and behavior to "entice" the child to engage. This method relies on the power of the intrinsic motivation of social engagement. It is thought that the social engagement promoted by Floortime will motivate the child to progress and learn.

The Hanen Centre: This is an online center that provides many resources for professionals, predominantly speech pathologists, who then integrate the Hanen methods into their therapy. Hanen methods focus on the adult-child interaction to build social, language, and play skills. The Hanen Centre offers parent education workshops, many educational materials for parents and professionals, and professional training for speech pathologists.

Naturalistic Developmental Behavioral Interventions

Naturalistic developmental behavioral interventions (NDBIs) integrate developmental approaches with behavioral principles. They are taught within a natural environment using natural or intrinsic rewards. For instance, if the child is working on making requests, the lesson is structured with a desired outcome that serves to reinforce successful communication. If the child seeks a favorite toy and, while engaging with the adult, communicates this desire, then achieving access to this preferred object serves to reinforce the desired skill. These interventions focus on skills that involve social engagement and reciprocal interaction, and therapy takes place during everyday activities and play. The adult and the child take turns leading the interaction.

Early Start Denver Model (ESDM): The ESDM is the most successfully studied NDBI. The ESDM is a therapy for children aged 12 to 48 months. The focus of the therapy is on building relationships. Play is used to encourage interaction and communication. Randomized controlled trials have demonstrated positive and lasting effects on social communication and play. These methods have been successful in the classroom and in parent-led intervention, and they are available for many therapists and educators to integrate into their work. Free parent webinars are available as well.

Pivotal response therapy (PRT): PRT is a child-centered therapy that focuses on teaching a child through motivating everyday play and activities. Specific skills of social communication are targeted, such as social initiation, response to others, and self-regulation. Pivotal response therapy is used by many ABA therapists.

Joint Attention, Symbolic Play, Engagement and Regulation (JASPER): JASPER is a play-based therapy that teaches social communication skills (joint attention, imitation, and play) to young children. This method is taught by educators, therapists, and parents.

Preschool Autism Communication Trial (PACT): PACT focuses on the parent-child dyad through video-assisted teaching. The parent is taught how to support social engagement and communication by analyzing videos of their interaction to find opportunities for teaching, modeling, and prompting social engagement and communication.

Enhanced milieu teaching (EMT): In EMT, the parent is taught to use the child's interests and initiations to teach conversational skills in everyday play and interaction. The strategies can be used during daily routines throughout the day.

Other Therapies

Augmentative and alternative communication (AAC): Many children and adults on the spectrum have significant motor planning dysfunctions and/or apraxia making the production and imitation of vocal sounds challenging. In these cases, the introduction of an alternative approach to communication becomes imperative while the child is doing therapy. Individuals on the spectrum may be minimally verbal or nonspeaking and benefit from a referral for alternative forms of communication (speech-generating devices [SGDs], American Sign Language [ASL], and/or the PECS).

The public school system has specialists who provide assessments and required AAC equipment. It is necessary for the pediatric primary care clinician to know which speech pathologists in their community are certified or fluent in the use of the AAC equipment or SGDs. Some schools and therapists recommend the introduction of the PECS or ASL first, before introducing computer-based software. Rarely are these 2 communication systems used as a primary form of communication. The PECS is cumbersome, and ASL involves motor planning skills that many children on the spectrum struggle with. American Sign Language is limited in utility because so few individuals in the population are fluent in its use. Many other communication specialists recommend beginning with speech-generating technology. Parents may have concern that a child will become dependent on a communication device and not learn to speak; however, research demonstrates that the use of an SGD is motivating to a child and allows the child to progress, communicate, and be successful while they are working on the oral expression of communication.

The software for these digital communication devices teaches children to use and build language in the way in which it typically develops, by teaching core language. Core language is the basic language needed in everyday interaction. The system chosen should be flexible and allow for easy progression in vocabulary, word combination, and goals as the child's ability increases. The communication applications should be placed onto a tablet that is available to the child at all times. Further, the tablet should not have access to games or the internet, as this may distract the child from using the tablet for communication purposes. Schools or private therapists will choose a software product such as Proloquo2Go or Language Acquisition through Motor Planning (LAMP) Words for Life, which are text-to-speech generating and therefore model the speech desired for the child. Communication software is customized for each individual so the symbols provided are appropriate for their level and may advance and be modified as they make progress. LAMP Words for Life also provides the individual with the ability to communicate independently through a touch screen of images, letters, or words. With this method, the individual initially learns to use words, builds functional vocabulary, and learns to build phrases, and, later, sentences, to communicate their wants, needs, and ideas by pressing buttons. This same device can easily be converted to spell words and communicate by using complete sentences. LAMP Words for Life uses the visual strength and memory of the individual while addressing the dysfunctions in motor skills and difficulties in social engagement to create spontaneous communication.

Occupational therapy (OT): OT has many applications for the autistic child. Occupational therapists may evaluate and address motor planning dysfunctions, delays in self-help skills, fine motor delays, sensory processing difficulties, and attentional and emotional dysregulation. Occupational therapists are especially skilled at assisting parents with many of the behavioral challenges that young children on the spectrum experience. They use curricula such as The Zones of Regulation to teach self-awareness and self-regulation in children at home and in the school. The Zones of Regulation is a curriculum that is used to teach children skills to self-regulate. The OT and/or educator identify triggers for a child's dysregulation and teach the child how to use tools independently to regulate. Some OT providers offer group therapy to work on social skills and play and may use available curricula to assist with these skills. These curricula may include *You Are a Social Detective! Explaining Social Thinking to Kids,* 2nd Edition; the Social Thinking curriculum; or, to teach executive function skills, the Unstuck and On Target curriculum.

When assessing for possible sensory challenges, the OT makes recommendations for adaptations to the environment to support the child. Occupational therapists are often skilled at evaluating the contributions of behavioral reinforcers in the environment. The OT can be helpful in guiding the adaptation of the child's environment to support their needs and avoid the reinforcement of behaviors that are not constructive.

Rapid Prompting Method (RPM), also known as Spelling to Communicate: Is a facilitated form of communication. The American Speech-Language-Hearing Association (ASHA) specifically warns against this type of therapy because of the reliance on an adult to prompt for its use. ASHA has stated that there are no reliable data to support this therapy. Despite ASHA's warning, RPM has been a very popular therapy among some families, and discussions with families about therapy methods offer the primary care clinician an opportunity to advise against its use.

In this method, a child is taught to spell by using a letter board while the facilitator provides physical prompts to the child. The RPM is a rapid-paced method using prompting to engage and teach a child to communicate ideas. This method seeks to address the underlying dysfunction in motor planning to allow a child to express their cognitive abilities and relies on an adult to hold and facilitate the communication spelling boards.

Social skills training: There are many tools available for teaching social skills. These tools are used by the gamut of specialists who work with the autistic child and are often available in private therapy and school settings. The Social Thinking methods (www.socialthinking.com) are widely used in schools to teach children older than 4 years how to understand the social world and support relationship. For older adolescents, the Program for the Education and Enrichment of Relational Skills (PEERS) is a certified evidence-based program that is available at many private centers both in person and on the internet. PEERS has documented efficacy in teaching many functional skills to adolescents. The PEERS curriculum breaks down social interaction into teachable steps, demonstrating to adolescents behaviors that are seen in successful social interactions.

It should be noted that it is not always expected or desirable to encourage the autistic child to aim to mimic the skills of their non-autistic peers. It can be extremely stressful for some on the spectrum to make eye contact or be expected to integrate with their peers. In all situations, peers and society should be encouraged to learn to understand and adapt their expectations of the autistic individual while appreciating their unique skills and strengths.

Speech therapy: Speech services offered for the autistic child are extremely varied from one practitioner to the next. It is important to clarify what the therapy goals are when referring a child: articulation, social engagement, use of words to make requests, expansion of core vocabulary, literacy skills, play, or assessment for augmentative forms of communication. The finding that many behavioral challenges arise from inadequate communication is a core principle of and motivation for beginning speech therapy. Traditionally, a speech pathologist may assist with vocalizations, word production, and articulation. Many children on the spectrum do struggle with the mechanics of vocalization, but all children will struggle in varying degrees with the core features of autism: social engagement, play, and functional communication. In the context of autism, the speech pathologist can be an essential member of the team who assists the parent with play and engagement in the home and teaches the use of words to make requests, narrate actions, respond to others in conversation, and build fundamental skills. Speech pathologists may use augmentative forms of communication when applicable. The speech pathologist approach to teaching communication is built on teaching the core vocabulary that a person requires to successfully communicate.

TEACCH: TEACCH is a method that relies on structured learning in an organized physical environment with a predictable sequence of activities. In the classroom, a variety of tools are used, such as visual schedules, flexible routines, and systems for choosing activities, to optimize the success of the autistic child. The TEACCH method is not widely available, although individual components such as the visual schedules are.

Practical Factors Influencing Choice of Intervention

There are many intervention methodologies available for the autistic child. Some are specific to autism and evidence based and others are based on approaches that have been used for children with a variety of developmental disorders. In practicality, choices are limited by which options are available through and covered by insurance. For most families, this means working with the options provided within the special education system, speech and occupational therapies, and ABA. Other therapies discussed may be available through academic centers or in different regions of the world. The pediatric primary care clinician should be knowledgeable about the choices within their community so they can have an educated discussion with families about their therapy options. As illustrated in the case vignette, individualizing recommendations based on the strengths and needs of the child guides the choices recommended. Ultimately, the clinician's recommendations are balanced with the family's needs and capabilities in choosing therapy. Parents have valid instincts about the philosophy and the educational culture to know whether each is consistent with their priorities for their child. The quality of the fit between therapist and family preferences and culture is as important in determining outcomes as the recommendations made based on research data. The collaboration that occurs will encourage the family to embrace the process and maximize the outcome of each method being taught.

CASE VIGNETTE: CONCLUSION

The primary care clinician raises the possibility that Rohan requires more individualized support to address his task avoidance and work on flexibility, social engagement, and language pragmatics. The clinician discusses that his behaviors in school and at home are worsening most likely because he is successful at avoiding tasks he does not like. As a result, his disruptive behaviors are being reinforced by their consequences. The clinician notes that his lack of social engagement and progressive resistance to directions and tasks are affecting his progress. Both his parents work full-time and see that his skills of independence are not progressing at home. He does not consistently use the toilet, declines to dress, and struggles with transitions throughout the day. His parents are not available to take him to multiple therapies throughout the day and do not feel they are capable of integrating these therapies into his everyday activities. They choose an integrated and intensive day therapy program that is covered by insurance. Together, the parents and primary care clinician decide that Rohan is best suited for a center-based, full-time applied behavior analysis (ABA) program through which he will benefit from a one-on-one therapist and the opportunity for social engagement with peers. The clinician reviews the criteria that the parents should use to select a quality service provider that will assist with the kindergarten transition and IEP planning. The family explores several options and selects the center with a location and hours that work for them. The family additionally expresses that they appreciate the diversity represented by the staff and families at the center and that they appreciate the importance placed on collaboration with the family. Rohan is withdrawn from the county-based special education class. The family will meet with the IEP team at the school in the spring of the following year to discuss kindergarten planning. Personnel from the ABA center will assist with planning and transition.

Clinical Pearls

- Research indicates that autism-specific manualized evidence-based approaches result in significant developmental progress compared to the broader EI services that are generally available in many communities.
- The intervention program should be comprehensive and involve at least 20 hours of autism-specific programming per week. These hours include the time a trained parent works with the child.
- Therapy should target all developmental domains that are relevant or underdeveloped or lagging for a particular child. These may include social-emotional development, behavioral regulation, executive function skills, functional communication, motor skills, adaptive skills, cognitive abilities, safety, and behavioral health.
- Therapy should include a parent training component.
- Coordination of treatment goals and methods should occur across settings or services.
- The ultimate goal of therapy is to promote inclusion or place the child into the least restrictive environment.

References

Cannon L, Kenworthy L, Alexander KC, Werner MA, Anthony L. *Unstuck and On Target: An Executive Function Curriculum to Improve Flexibility, Planning, and Organization.* 2nd ed. Brookes Publishing Co; 2021

Evidence-based practices. The National Professional Development Center on Autism Spectrum Disorder. Accessed March 2, 2026. https://autismpdc.fpg.unc.edu/ebps

Hyman SL, Levy SE, Myers SM, et al; American Academy of Pediatrics Council on Children With Disabilities and Section on Developmental and Behavioral Pediatrics. Identification, evaluation, and management of children with autism spectrum disorder. *Pediatrics.* 2020;145(1):e20193447 PMID: 31843864 doi: 10.1542/peds.2019-3447

Pickles A, Le Couteur A, Leadbitter K, et al. Parent-mediated social communication therapy for young children with autism (PACT): long-term follow-up of a randomised controlled trial. *Lancet.* 2016;388(10059):2501–2509 PMID: 27793431 doi: 10.1016/S0140-6736(16)31229-6

Rogers SJ, Estes A, Lord C, et al. A multisite randomized controlled two-phase trial of the Early Start Denver Model compared to treatment as usual. *J Am Acad Child Adolesc Psychiatry.* 2019;58(9):853–865 PMID: 30768394 doi: 10.1016/j.jaac.2019.01.004

Sandbank M, Bottema-Beutel K, Crowley S, et al. Project AIM: autism intervention meta-analysis for studies of young children. *Psychol Bull.* 2020;146(1):1–29 PMID: 31763860 doi: 10.1037/bul0000215

Sandbank M, Bottema-Beutel K, Woynaroski T. Intervention recommendations for children with autism in light of a changing evidence base. *JAMA Pediatr.* 2021;175(4):341–342 PMID: 33165523 doi: 10.1001/jamapediatrics.2020.4730

CHAPTER

9

Autism and Behavioral Challenges: Why They Occur and How to Approach Them

CASE VIGNETTE 1

Bryan is an 11-year-old child who is well-known to his pediatric primary care clinician. He received a diagnosis of autism in preschool and attended elementary school in a self-contained autism-centered classroom. He was placed into some general education classes in his areas of academic strength. During the latter years of elementary school, Bryan was diagnosed with co-occurring attention-deficit/hyperactivity disorder (ADHD) and had a positive response to the regular use of psychostimulants. He had done well until the fall of his first year in middle school, when he presents to his primary care clinician for repeated suspensions for behavioral outbursts and acts of aggression. Bryan's parents feel embarrassed and overwhelmed by his behavior, so they consult with the primary care clinician to discuss whether his ADHD medications are still working. The teachers are surprised by Bryan's behavior and have been sending him home for escalating behavior. His parents have been punishing Bryan for behavior they find unacceptable and seek guidance from the primary care clinician.

Prior chapters have discussed that individuals on the autism spectrum by definition have delays in areas of communication, social engagement, and processing of sensory stimuli and have restricted and repetitive behaviors and interests. Given the nature of these attributes, one can imagine how the world can at times be confusing, overwhelming, and anxiety producing to an individual with difficulties and differences in coping abilities and the ability to communicate. The frustration that may result often leads to behaviors that evolve from fight-or-flight types of responses to perceived threats or stress, as they would for any human. The pediatric primary care clinician may be consulted by families when these behaviors occur. Alternatively, the school may refer the child for a medical evaluation, or behavioral specialists may want a medical opinion. Although these challenges are unlikely to be noticed in a highly structured setting such as a primary care office, review of a child's care plan should involve addressing these types of behavioral concerns and understanding the resources and strategies for support.

Definition of Behavioral Challenges

Behavioral challenges are typically defined as disruptive irritability, tantrums, or acts of aggression, all of which are likely to cause harm to individuals, property, or self. When behaviors interfere with a child's ability to engage with others, learn, or perform daily tasks, or if they put someone's well-being at risk, a systematic approach is required. A 2016 meta-analysis of available research data provides practice parameters for managing behavioral challenges (referred to as "irritability or problem behaviors" in the meta-analysis) and includes an excellent algorithm for decision-making (**Figure 9.1**). This approach to managing such challenges will be addressed in this chapter. **Box 9.1** lists helpful resources available for both parents and professionals on the topic of addressing behavioral challenges.

Constructive change for children and adolescents on the autism spectrum requires a systematic approach to understanding why these behaviors occur, as they would in any child, so accommodations can be made to support the child or adolescent. At times, when professionals in the medical setting approach behaviors that are disruptive to one's functioning or others' space (referred to in this chapter as *disruptive behaviors* for easier reading), they look for behavioral strategies or medication to manage, suppress, or extinguish behaviors without seeking to understand the environmental triggers and areas of developmental need that may precipitate the behaviors. As has been discussed in earlier chapters, individuals on the spectrum may demonstrate impulsivity and have difficulties with regulating emotion, communicating, and understanding abstract concepts. They may have

BOX 9.1 Behavioral Challenges: Resources for Parents and Professionals

- Autism Speaks, Challenging Behaviors Tool Kit: www.autismspeaks.org/tool-kit/challenging-behaviors-tool-kit
- Baker J. *No More Meltdowns: Positive Strategies for Managing and Preventing Out-of-Control Behavior.* Future Horizons; 2008
- Kuypers LM. *The Zones of Regulation: A Curriculum Designed to Foster Self-Regulation and Emotional Control.* Think Social Publishing; 2011
- Sesame Street, Monster Meditation: www.youtube.com/watch?v=3EKPfQYi7GQ
- Wrightslaw special education and law advocacy: www.wrightslaw.com/idea

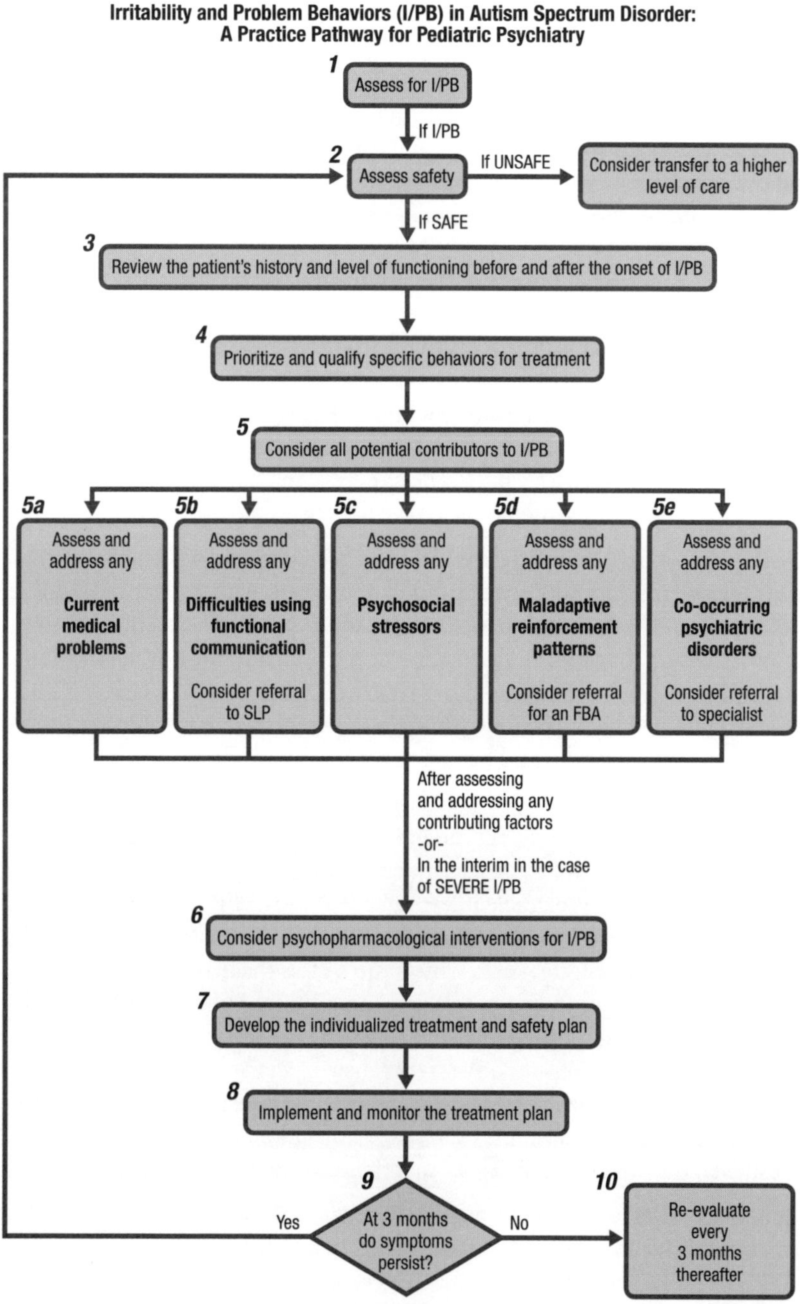

Figure 9.1. Irritability and Problem Behavior in Autism Spectrum Disorder: A Practice Pathway for Pediatric Psychiatry

SLP indicates speech-language pathologist.

Reproduced from McGuire K, Fung LK, Hagopian L, et al. Irritability and problem behavior in autism spectrum disorder: a practice pathway for pediatric primary care. *Pediatrics.* 2016;137(suppl 2):S136–S148.

inflexible thinking and may not be able to take the perspective of others. When routines change, when a substitute teacher has different expectations, when a new lesson presents challenges, or when the use of idioms or more complex and abstract language confuses an autistic child, the child may be challenged beyond their ability. A peer may do something that an individual on the spectrum may find wrong or unacceptable without having the ability to take the perspective of that peer. Individuals on the spectrum often have very literal interpretations of rules and may not be able to tolerate when others do not follow rules. Their emotional responses might appear out of proportion to the triggering event. These contributors explain why behavioral challenges are commonplace for those with an autism diagnosis. The focus of this chapter is to understand these behavioral differences, to identify where the triggers for behavioral challenges lie, and to focus support on making adaptations to the environment and teaching where skill-related areas of need are identified. Approaches will vary from teaching concrete skill sets to putting systems into place to support the child as they learn to adapt to different circumstances and environments.

A classic example of how skill-related areas of need can lead to behavioral challenges is the interpretation of speed limits on the road. Although speed limit signs exist to represent the law, most people understand there is an acceptable range of variation. The sign may set the speed limit at 55 mph, but most drivers will understand they can drive 5 to 10 miles above this limit without a high risk of being approached by the police. The individual on the spectrum may interpret this guidance in a very literal fashion and become upset if anyone drives above or below this suggested speed.

The autistic child may become argumentative, explosive, or even aggressive when feeling challenged or provoked. This behavior occurs regularly with many social rules that have a range of tolerable interpretations. Most children may understand this range, but the autistic child tends to abide literally by the rules. Most children will understand they can speak in a whisper in a class that has a "no talking" rule, but the autistic child may interpret this rule literally and forbid all talking at all times. A transition might be asked of the autistic child before they feel satisfied they have completed the previous task. A teacher may expect a response in a specific time frame that exceeds the slower processing speed of the autistic child. The autistic child may state direct observations, such as "I don't like your haircut" or "Your breath smells bad," without awareness that these comments could cause offense.

The autistic child may need to be taught the rules of the social world in a very systematic way. It cannot be taken for granted that a child on the spectrum understands how to take the perspective of others or how their own behavior affects others. Temple Grandin, a prominent spokesperson for autism, has discussed her need to create different categories of rules as she learned to navigate the social world: those that can never be broken, those that are polite and result in people feeling good, and, last, those that are illegal but not bad and can at times be broken.

She created lists of these rules and approached the social world in this type of logical fashion to learn how to be more successful. In many of her books, she describes how parents and professionals are obligated to teach these social rules to children on the spectrum to give them the structure they need to know how to behave in different settings. It is this understanding of the cognitive and social differences that children on the spectrum experience that will inform the pediatric clinician's understanding of behavioral challenges for these children.

The ideal approach to behavioral challenges is to recognize that the behavior associated with them exists for a reason, or what is called a *function*. The behavior may be a call for help rather than defiance. It is the responsibility of the professionals working with the child to understand the reasons behind the behaviors and identify the underlying life skills to be taught. This approach helps the child adapt to the demands of more typical experiences and experience fewer instances of emotional dysregulation. The goal of a professional in approaching such behaviors is to carefully collect data about the child so the professional and parents can learn and apply new strategies to teach the child more adaptive responses and make the necessary adjustments to routines that will prevent the occurrence of the disruptive behaviors. In most cases, a child will demonstrate improved behavior if there is more predictability in their environment, an understanding of expectations and procedures, a safety plan, and an emphasis on teaching skills of self-regulation, communication, and self-determination.

Assessing Safety

If the autistic child or anyone else is at risk for harm because of the child's behavioral challenges, an immediate crisis plan is required. This may require calling a crisis intervention hotline, taking the child to an emergency department (only if the risk for escalation is considered high), or placing the child into a more restrictive/therapeutic environment with a higher level of trained supervision in the school setting until a successful behavior plan is assembled. It is beyond the scope of this guidebook or the role of the pediatric primary care clinician to teach de-escalation strategies, but advising families on expected procedures can be extremely helpful when families are coping with issues regarding safety and escalating, dysregulated behaviors.

When the pediatric primary care clinician reviews the case of a child on the autism spectrum whose behavior is disruptive or creating behavioral challenges, it is important to ensure that those involved in everyday care of the child do not attempt to teach the child a lesson, ask the child to apologize, or reiterate the injustice that has resulted from the situation while the child is demonstrating dysregulated behavior. It can be helpful to suggest to the teacher, parent, or therapist to simply walk with the child or be physically present, with the goal of de-escalating or preventing further disruption. This is a temporary step until a plan can be put into place. Physical proximity between an adult and the child may provide a calming influence, and the use of empathy can be effective in diverting a meltdown; "I understand this is really hard for you" or "I see you are trying very hard" are examples of this type of shared empathy that can be effective. The adult should avoid threats or physical constraints and usher the child, if possible, to a quiet place. During extreme outbursts, it is safer to remove everyone else from the room rather than attempt to move a child whose behavior is escalating.

Describing the Behavior

To understand a behavior, a thorough description of the behavior and circumstances is needed. The parent, with the assistance of the teachers, should describe in objective language the behaviors they are observing. The primary care clinician may need to reach out to the professionals caring for the child to obtain this information. The clinician should ask questions to obtain additional details, and if the descriptions include indications of judgment or the use of presumed diagnoses, the clinician should advocate for more objective details. Often adjectives such as "lazy," "defiant," or "ADHD-like" will be used by a parent or teacher before anyone has enough information. The pediatric primary care clinician needs to know how often the behaviors occur, how intense they are, how long they last, and where and under what circumstances they occur.

Clinicians use the following **FINDS** acronym to determine the effects of a behavior:

F**requency:** How often is the behavior occurring?

I**ntensity:** Describe the behavior in detail to determine if there is risk for personal or physical harm.

N**umber of associated circumstances:** Collect information about the number of precipitating associated circumstances.

D**uration:** How long does the behavior last?

S**etting:** Where and in what settings does it occur?

Collecting this information elucidates the extent of the behavior's effects and the related challenges and determines next steps to identify the underlying skill sets that need to be addressed.

Understanding the Behavior's Function

When disruptive behaviors occur recurrently or predictably, it is likely they are being triggered and/or reinforced by the child's environment. This presents an opportunity for proactive planning using behavioral principles to effect change. Recurring disruptive behaviors become predictable because they reflect an underlying developmental challenge and are reinforced by the consequences that occur. These recurring behaviors tend to fall into one of 4 categories as summarized in **Box 9.2**.

BOX 9.2 Why Disruptive Behaviors Recur in Children on the Autism Spectrum

Disruptive behaviors that recur have the following underlying motivations:

- To avoid a demand or a situation
- To gain access to someone or something
- To secure attention from others
- To either avoid or engage with a sensory stimulus

A child may avoid a demand placed on them that they do not understand, that is too challenging or overwhelming, or that they do not feel motivated to accomplish. If they protest or elope and are able to successfully avoid the demand, the behavior is likely to continue. If a child prefers to be with a certain person, to be in a different place, or to engage in a specific activity and the escape behavior allows them to gain that access, the behavior is likely to continue. If the child seeks and is successful at securing attention from others because of a behavioral response, the behavior is likely to continue. Last, many individuals on the autism spectrum may seek out a specific sensory experience (eg, putting their hands into materials, putting objects into their mouth, running, jumping, climbing, singing, spinning, getting outside). Alternatively, they may seek to avoid sensory experiences that are noxious to them (eg, hand driers or flushers in public restrooms, loud noises, a specific experience, a person, an image). They may run to avoid the experience and, if successful at avoiding it, will likely continue to exhibit this behavior until they are taught ways to cope with the trigger or the trigger is adjusted.

What Is a Functional Behavioral Assessment?

To understand the function of a behavior that is felt to significantly and negatively affect a child's ability to engage in daily activities, a functional behavioral assessment (FBA) must be performed. This might be initiated by the pediatric primary care clinician with the parent in the office, through a discussion that reviews the behavior and elucidates its function or cause. In most situations, a more formalized collection of data by school personnel or by a behavioral specialist is required. The Individuals with Disabilities Act requires that a child receiving special education services who has behavior that "impairs their ability to function in the classroom" is entitled to a formal FBA within the school setting.

The purpose of the FBA is to better understand what function a disruptive behavior is serving for the child or why the behavior is occurring. The goal is to identify triggers to the observed behavior and infer what skills need to be taught. The consequences of the behavior clarify how the environment is involved and possibly reinforcing the behavior.

All FBAs use the following **ABC** acronym for collecting information about the function of the behavior associated with behavioral challenges:

Antecedents: In this type of assessment, the observational data collected describes the antecedents or triggers that precede and seem related to the behavior. It should be noted that antecedents do not always occur immediately before the trigger, so a more thorough history may be necessary. For example, at times a poor night's sleep or an argument at home the night before may have been the triggering event. Antecedents help clinicians understand skill-related areas that suggest the need for supportive strategies. Is the demand reasonable for this child? Has something occurred before a demand to make the child less likely to be successful, such as a challenging transition or interaction? Was the child avoiding a demand, trying to gain access to something, or attempting to secure the attention of someone? Was there an interaction that was upsetting the child?

***B*ehavior:** The professional performing the FBA collects detailed information from a parent or an educator or directly observes and describes the behavior in clear, complete, and objective language. They should avoid making a diagnosis and simply describe the behavioral changes observed so anyone receiving the report has a clear idea of what has occurred. Documentation of the FINDS is essential.

Consequences: The reactions of adults and children to the behavior and resulting events help the consultant performing the FBA understand how the consequences of that behavior serve to reinforce its function. Is the child receiving some attention as a result? Is the child successfully avoiding a task or gaining access to something they are seeking? These outcomes could inadvertently reinforce the behavior by providing secondary gain. In summary, it is imperative that any consequences put into place for a behavior do not inadvertently reinforce the behavior by allowing avoidance of the triggering demand.

The following case vignette illustrates how an FBA can elucidate the reason for the behavior associated with behavioral challenges and help the care team focus on skill-related areas of need that require teaching.

CASE VIGNETTE 2

USING FUNCTIONAL BEHAVIORAL ANALYSIS TO DETERMINE THE CAUSE OF THE BEHAVIOR ASSOCIATED WITH BEHAVIORAL CHALLENGES

An elementary school–aged child has a history of recurring episodes of fleeing or eloping from the classroom to avoid schoolwork. The child has repeatedly been sent to the principal's office or suspended for discipline without any improvement. The parents have been notified and bring their concern to their pediatric primary care clinician. This behavior occurs regularly and with increasing frequency and is significantly and negatively affecting the child's academic performance. The teachers and parents do not identify clinically significant symptoms of ADHD. The progression of the behavior suggests that it serves a function for the child. The individualized education program (IEP) team requests an FBA and learns that the classroom has transitioned to preparing for an exam and that relevant material is heavily based on abstract language skills. The child is struggling in this area of language comprehension, becomes very anxious, misses important instruction, and becomes restless before running out of the room. He thus successfully avoids a difficult task but, as a result, is falling further behind, which is compounding his anxiety. The behavior becomes progressively more self-fulfilling and is reinforced by the response of the school. An appropriate response should include assistance with the language-based learning in this lesson by providing more educational supports, as well as breaking lessons down into concrete, visually based instruction. A visual schedule with a positive behavioral incentive is indicated. The teachers become more aware that the child is struggling with the classroom tasks and does not yet know how to communicate that he is overwhelmed and needs help. A plan to teach the child self-calming skills and work on the child's ability to express his feelings and use problem-solving strategies to deal with challenges would lead both to resolution of the behavior and to the development of more optimal skills.

Essential Components of a Behavioral Intervention Plan

Once the function of a behavior is understood, a behavioral intervention plan (BIP) can be created. The behavioral specialist will articulate the specific replacement behaviors or skills that will need to be taught so the child has more successes and the behavioral challenges recede. The BIP will include the specific behavior goals and will address the factors that are serving as reinforcers. Additionally, the BIP will specify how skills will be taught, detail which accommodations are needed, and delineate a plan for monitoring progress. It is helpful for the pediatric primary care clinician to advise parents on when to request an FBA and what to expect of the FBA and BIP. The FBA and BIP will be documents that are added to a child's educational plan and should be accessible for parents to bring for review with their pediatric clinician.

A BIP may include assurance that teacher demands are clear, appropriate, and concise while implementing visual supports and a predictable schedule of demands. In some cases, restructuring the environment so there are fewer distractions is indicated. The child may need to be taught specific skills such as how to take turns, ask for help or a break, engage in a nonpreferred activity, or transition from an activity they like to another they prefer less. The team will determine whether the demands being placed on the child are realistic. A guiding principle is that 80% of the demands of the day should be easy for a child to complete. The remaining 20% of demands will require effort, focus, and learned new skills. Often the school will lessen demands when a child is struggling, put a behavior plan into place, and then increase expectations once there is improvement in the child's ability to demonstrate the desired behaviors. Rather than simply remove the demands, it is preferable to adjust the expectations so the child can meet them successfully. Over time, as the child's ability to meet expectations is established with the appropriate amount of support, the demands can again be increased. The team should establish appropriate behavioral incentives, such as including the child's preferred interests in a lesson plan. The short case vignettes that follow exemplify some of these concepts.

CASE VIGNETTE 3

INAPPROPRIATE EXPECTATIONS

Jada is a high school student on the autism spectrum who was told by her teacher that she has symptoms of ADHD. She has never been formally evaluated for this diagnosis. She has been practicing arithmetic calculations repeatedly at home and through an after-school program. Because of her success with these calculations, her parents have assumed that her math skills are at grade level and feel strongly that she participate in general education math in high school. When Jada comes to her primary care clinician for her health supervision visit, her parents report that she has had a profound increase in repetitive rocking, hair pulling, and disruptive vocalizations. Jada's parents are perplexed and ask if she might benefit from being treated with ADHD medication. On review of Jada's psychological testing, it is apparent that her math concepts are in the very low or deficient range, despite her strength with calculations. Behavioral observations in the classroom reveal that her behavior is both a manifestation of the anxiety and an attempt to self-soothe, which have developed in response to academic demands that exceed her abilities. Once the demands are adjusted to her abilities, these behaviors improve dramatically. The concern for possible ADHD is not pursued.

CASE VIGNETTE 4

USING THE CHILD'S INTERESTS

Ishan is a 7-year-old autistic boy who struggles to attend to academic lessons. His teachers know that one of his favorite activities is studying catalogs of automobiles. His parents bring catalogs of cars for the teachers to use. The teachers find it highly effective to reward Ishan's attention to nonpreferred academic study with allotments of time with his catalogs. In addition, lessons are modified so his reading and math work have content that includes cars, car manufacturer logos, and the details of each model. Ishan's teachers have included stories and created math problems that involve images and descriptions of cars. The teachers find that Ishan feels more motivated to attend to his lessons and that his academic performance strengthens when his interests are included.

The final step in putting together a successful behavior plan is assessing what adaptive behaviors need to be taught to the child. The pediatric primary care clinician, as well as the parent and behavioral specialist, can have input into what skill-related areas of need lead to the behavioral challenge. One such area of need in development may be communication. A child on the spectrum may have strengths in vocabulary but struggle to use the language to identify and get their needs met. Some of these children will need to be taught how to use their language in this context or use an augmentative form of communication. With other children, behavioral challenges are more related to the atypical features of autism such as sensory vulnerabilities, restricted and repetitive behaviors, difficulties with social awareness, and/or executive function skills. Many children will require a focus on teaching specific skills to regulate emotions. **Box 9.3** summarizes areas that are likely to be triggers for behaviors and that should be considered as the BIP is constructed.

BOX 9.3 Skill-Related Areas of Need That Are Often the Root of Behavioral Challenges

- **Transitions:** Does the child struggle to flexibly transition or meet social demands?
- **Communication needs:** Does the child struggle to communicate when they need help or a break? Is there a clear plan for teaching communication skills? Would the child benefit from use of an augmentative and alternative communication device and consultation (refer to the Other Therapies section in Chapter 8, Evidence-Based Supports and Services)? Often communication is the skill-related area of need underlying a behavioral challenge.
- **Demands:** Are the expectations of the classroom and the social interactions reasonable for this child? Can they easily accomplish 80% of the demands? Do demands need to be broken down into individual steps? Does the child need more one-on-one assistance to receive encouragement, to get prompts for next steps, or to effectively use strategies being taught? Are instructions clear and are visuals used to reinforce these instructions, encourage independence, and appeal to the child's strength in visual learning?
- **Sensory features:** Are there sensory experiences that interfere with the child's success? Is the child distracted, fearful, avoidant, or becoming dysregulated when exposed to a specific sensory experience? This response happens often in places such as the bathroom, gymnasiums, or playgrounds, or during events such as school assemblies, group experiences, or birthday celebrations.
- **Self-regulation skills:** Does the behavior plan include teaching self-calming strategies? Is self-regulation built into many aspects of teaching? Many individuals on the autism spectrum will struggle with self-regulation of moods and attention and benefit from a comprehensive program in this area. The Zones of Regulation is one such program (https://zonesofregulation.com). In this curriculum, a child learns to identify when they are regulated, when they are becoming dysregulated, and when they have reached a state of dysregulation. Then they are provided with a toolkit of skills to use independently to help return themselves to a regulated attentional state.
- **Strength-based teaching:** Is the curriculum adapted to encourage engagement, ability to meet behavioral expectations, and success throughout the day by using the child's strengths? Are the child's preferred interests included in the teachings? Does the curriculum call on the child's developmental strengths and encouragement in the classroom?

Continued on next page

BOX 9.3 *(continued)*

- **Social understanding:** Does the child have an appropriate understanding of the rules of social functioning required to be successful? What specific social skills need to be taught? It is important to remember that children on the spectrum struggle to take the perspective of others. They may feel motivated to engage with peers but not have the skills to do so successfully. Often a comment made by the autistic individual may be based on the truth but hurtful in its effect. The autistic child's need to enforce rules that are being broken by typically developing peers can precipitate conflict or isolation and alienate peers.
- **Executive function skills:** Do accommodations need to be put into place to support the child in staying organized and on task? Most individuals on the spectrum benefit from a predictable and organized environment that has clear routines and is free of multiple distracters. Having instruction broken down into steps and using visual schedules may be more helpful than relying on lengthy verbal descriptions. Sometimes a simple visual representation or a model of the goal of a lesson will be highly instructive.
- **Positive behavioral supports:** The use of positive behavioral supports strengthens relationships and an individual's sense of competence. This can enhance behavioral responses to situational demands. Positive behavior programs focus on times when the child is on task and engaged in constructive behaviors and emphasize reinforcement of these behaviors. Reinforcers can be as simple as a comment ("I see you are working hard") or a warm response from an adult, or they may require an extrinsic reward system. Too often, adults expect children to engage constructively and do not reinforce their successes.

Children requiring a focus on emotional regulation may need to be taught specific strategies to learn how to independently identify triggers for their behavior, their mood state, and specific strategies for self-calming. Some of the skills and strategies taught to promote self-regulation are

- Asking for help when overwhelmed or in need.
- Asking for a break when stressed.
- Using words to identify how one is feeling.
- Having a quiet place where one can engage in self-calming strategies. The quiet place can have sensory tools one finds soothing (eg, music, a book, a headset, a special blanket).
- Using meditation to self-calm.
- Practicing deep breathing exercises (eg, blowing a tissue, blowing bubbles, doing figure eight breathing, or doing other breathing exercises) (refer to deep breathing exercises available through the Children's Healthcare of Atlanta Strong4Life program: www.strong4life.com/en/emotional-wellness/coping/practicing-deep-breathing).
- Having a safety plan that includes keeping others safe and having a safe place where one can go and/or a special person whom one trusts to help support de-escalation.

Possible Medical Contributors

It is important to consider all possible contributors to behavioral challenges, including biological ones, before implementing a behavior plan. Even if they are not the primary cause, medical contributors are likely to exacerbate disruptive behavior and can certainly add to the resulting level of difficulty. The pediatric primary care clinician should focus on the identification and treatment of medical contributors to ameliorate symptoms and optimize the success of behavioral and educational therapies. The primary care clinician's role here is critical and may result in dramatic improvements. Potential medical contributors to behavioral challenges are described in **Box 9.4**. These are common pediatric differential diagnoses, but in the context of a child with a developmental condition, the threshold for consideration of these entities should be significantly lower. Several of these co-occurring conditions are more common and are discussed in more detail in Chapters 10, Diagnosing and Managing Co-Occurring Conditions; 11, Gastrointestinal Symptoms and Feeding Challenges; and 12, Insomnia: Identification and Interventions.

BOX 9.4 **Possible Medical Contributors to Behavioral Challenges**

- **Sleep deprivation** (refer to Chapter 12, Insomnia: Identification and Interventions): It is well-known that individuals with inadequate sleep can exhibit inattention, decreased academic performance, and increased disruptive behaviors.
- **Pain sources:** In addition to typical pain sources such as constipation, gastroesophageal reflux disease, and sinus or ear pressure, clinicians should consider dental pain and ensure that the child has routine preventive dental visits.
- **Gastrointestinal issues:** Constipation, celiac disease, eosinophilic esophagitis or gastroesophageal reflux disease, and toileting issues may manifest with exacerbation of underlying behavioral dysregulation. Because of a combination of poor communication skills and/or atypical sensory processing, individuals on the autism spectrum may not report specific symptoms of gastrointestinal disease.
- **Chronic respiratory symptoms:** Allergies, sinus congestion, and reactive airway disease may contribute to irritability, insomnia, and pain.
- **Irritation and skin issues:** Skin conditions such as atopic skin disease, eczema, pruritus, or hives can contribute to irritability and should be addressed aggressively.
- **Seizure disorders:** These disorders are more common in children on the spectrum and may manifest as a disruptive behavior, slow developmental progress, sleep interruption, or the exacerbation of preexisting conditions. A careful review of history and/or referral to a neurologist is indicated if there is concern.
- **Medication/stimulant adverse effects:** Clinicians should elicit a careful history of what the child is eating, what ingestions are possible, or what medications the child is taking. For example, selective serotonin reuptake inhibitors and stimulants are more likely to produce adverse effects such as irritability or "activation" in children and adolescents on the spectrum; thus, these medications should be started at very low doses and titrated up very slowly. In addition, exposure to caffeine-containing drinks should be considered.

Continued on next page

BOX 9.4 *(continued)*

- **Co-occurring behavioral health conditions:** Children and adolescents on the spectrum are at increased risk for attention-deficit/hyperactivity disorder, anxiety, depression, or irritability. These issues can be responsible for underlying struggles and internalizing or externalizing behaviors. The autistic child with significant externalizing behaviors should be screened for these possible behavioral health conditions by administering screening tools to parents, teachers, and the child (if appropriate). When the primary drive for the behavior appears related to a co-occurring mental health condition, referral and/or medication may be considered (refer to Chapter 13, Review of Pharmacotherapy and Complementary Interventions).
- **Communication delay:** Children on the spectrum are less likely to be effective communicators when expressing their emotions, asking for help, or solving problems. Children with communication delays of any type are at increased risk for behavioral challenges. The behavior plan will need to include teaching the necessary communication goals to support the child's interactions and performance. Additionally, referring the child for an assessment for an augmentative and alternative communication system may be indicated when verbal expression is limited.

Social Drivers of Health

As with any child, behavioral challenges can be the most obvious manifestation of environmental stressors. Stressors such as parental mental health condition or substance use, exposure to discord or violence, poverty, or harsh parenting practices can lead to emotional dysregulation and externalizing behaviors in all youth. Research literature and clinical experience demonstrate that factors that are destabilizing for all children can produce exaggerated responses in individuals with developmental conditions. **Box 9.5** lists environmental stressors that may be associated with behavioral challenges.

Follow-Up Plan

On completion of the process of an FBA, the team of professionals and parents better understand the child's behavioral challenges and the opportunities for educational support to ensure progress. The follow-up plan is an important component of the support. There should be a concrete plan for strategies and behavior goals. Teachers and other professionals involved in the child's care may require specific behavioral training and supervision to ensure consistency of behavioral strategies. Data should be collected to document the baseline function and subsequent response to strategies for both the disruptive behavior and the targeted skills being taught. This data should be tracked and reviewed by the

BOX 9.5 Possible Environmental Stressors Contributing to Behavioral Challenges

- **Adverse childhood experiences:** Adverse childhood experiences include those related to poverty, food insecurity, homelessness, exposure to violence or abuse, parental mental health challenges, significant familial stressors, or changes in the home environment.
- **Bullying:** Individuals with disabilities or neurodivergence, such as autism, are at increased risk for bullying. This is especially true for children on the spectrum who are very verbal and intelligent and receive services in a mainstream classroom with few support services.
- **Parental stress and harsh parenting practices:** Both these factors are predictors of behavioral challenges in children, and parents who experience stress or use harsh parenting techniques can benefit from referral for positive behavioral supports. There are many evidence-based parenting programs that are particularly useful in teaching parents strategies that reinforce positive behaviors and promote healthy parent-child relationships. Referrals for such programs can be very helpful. Programs and resources to support positive and effective parenting practices include Parent-Child Interaction Therapy, Triple P—Positive Parenting Program, or online training and resources such as the Mount Sinai Parenting Center (https://parenting.mountsinai.org), HealthySteps (www.healthysteps.org), Autism Speaks Challenging Behaviors Tool Kit (www.autismspeaks.org/tool-kit/challenging-behaviors-tool-kit), and *No More Meltdowns: Positive Strategies for Managing and Preventing Out-of-Control Behavior* by Jed Baker.
- **Poor fit between the child and their classroom environment:** At times, the education team will be called on to review the appropriateness of fit between a child, their peer group, supports available in the classroom, educational demands, and the skill set of the teaching team to determine whether a change in school or classroom should be considered.
- **Issues related to gender identity or sexuality:** Individuals on the spectrum are at increased risk for challenges around sexuality and gender identity. These can manifest as stress, anxiety, depression, and irritability and should be considered when evaluating possible causes of behavioral challenges.

behavioral specialist. Based on this data, it may be necessary to modify support as needed, ensuring fidelity of response with teachers. The progress evaluation should occur periodically as necessary. There should be a plan for communication with the parent(s), and the parent(s) may find it helpful to review progress with the team as well as independently with the pediatric primary care clinician.

If there is no improvement in the child's behavior, a parent has the right to request an independent educational evaluation at public expense whereby the child is evaluated by an outside consultant. The pediatric primary care clinician can be helpful in making these recommendations and supporting the parent through these requests. The outside professional will assess the behavior plan and the child's progress. Many parents choose to work with private behavioral therapists in addition to the process initiated by the school and then have these professionals attend regular progress or IEP meetings.

CASE VIGNETTE 1: CONCLUSION

Bryan had transitioned from a highly supervised, self-contained autism special education setting in elementary school to a less restrictive noncategorical placement in a new middle school and is engaging in disruptive behaviors during lunchtime. In this new setting, there has been opportunity for him to interact with typically developing peers for the first time. After the IEP team confers with a behavioral specialist and Bryan is observed in the lunchroom, it is discovered that Bryan has felt highly motivated to be with his peers and has approached them readily in the lunchroom with little structure or special education support. When engaging with his peers, Bryan is observed to speak repeatedly about his interests (air purifiers), and his peers not only appear uninterested but respond with annoyance. His peers have tried to ignore him, but when he persists in talking about his air purifier interests, some of his peers respond with hurtful comments. There is no adult available to supervise or support. Bryan's response is then to try harder to engage his peers. Bryan is observed to progress from being sad to becoming explosive and throwing objects as the responses of his peers become more insulting.

The IEP team has determined that the antecedents to Bryan's disruptive behaviors are his lack of success in constructively engaging his peers, despite his high level of social motivation. His peers' increasingly hurtful responses to his attempts to engage result in an escalation of his behaviors.

The BIP includes Bryan participating in a social skills program where learning focuses on turn taking in conversation while maintaining someone else's topic of conversation. In addition, a few of his peers are prepared to be available to model successful peer engagement, and because of their role as mentors, many of them become more invested in helping Bryan be successful. An adult is trained to be present in the lunchroom to support Bryan in finding opportunities to engage with his peers and prompt him to make constructive choices to keep his peers interested and engaged. The adult is able to offer redirection when there are struggles between Bryan and his peers and to use self-regulation strategies with Bryan.

Bryan and his parents are taught strategies for promoting and finding more opportunities to practice constructive peer engagement outside of school. They work on responding to others' comments, maintaining conversational topics, and observing the signs of others' responses to Bryan to guide his decisions. Bryan's parents find that he has progressed even further after they place him into a formal social skills class in his community.

The team meets periodically and reviews the data on Bryan's explosive behavior. Over time, the behavior resolves as there is constructive support for Bryan to be more successful in interaction and to learn to recognize and regulate his own emotional responses to others. In addition, drawing his peers into his learning is instrumental in motivating them to be more accepting and see the value of mentoring him. They begin to invite him to join them and even initiate some conversations about his interests.

Disruptive behaviors and behavioral challenges are a child's call for help when they are overwhelmed and unable to successfully meet expectations. These behaviors and challenges identify opportunities for support and learning and help inform the care team that a different approach is needed. The process of behavioral analysis is labor-intensive but can represent a chance to better understand the child and what strategies need to be implemented for the child to succeed. Behavioral analysis and support often identify opportunities for significant developmental progress. The involvement of the pediatric primary care clinician in this journey is vital, as they can assess the progress, identify potential accompanying conditions, and support the family in advocating for the best care practices.

Clinical Pearls

- Individuals on the autism spectrum are vulnerable to behavioral outbursts because of the nature of their developmental challenges. They may have insufficient coping skills, have limited ability to communicate, or may become anxious and/or overwhelmed by the demands of their social and educational worlds.
- A constructive approach to behavioral challenges requires a systematic approach to understand why the behavior occurs.
- Support should focus on teaching the skills needed for the child to be successful.
- Clinicians should use the FINDS (**f**requency, **i**ntensity, **n**umber of associated circumstances, **d**uration, and **s**etting) acronym to determine the extent of the behavior and its effects and be certain that the behavior has been objectively described.
- An FBA may be required to learn the function of a behavior by studying the antecedents to the behavior, what the behavior consists of, and the consequences of the behavior.
- After an FBA is completed, a BIP will be created and implemented to detail accommodations needed and to teach the child the skills required for success and growth.
- Clinicians should consider contributing and/or causative factors such as social drivers of health and medical conditions.
- The follow-up plan is key to ensuring that the behavior plan is effective.

References

Carbone PS, Farley M, Davis T. Primary care for children with autism. *Am Fam Physician.* 2010;81(4):453–460 PMID: 20148499

Grandin T. Learning social rules. Autism Asperger's Digest. January/February 2005. Accessed March 2, 2026. https://www.autismforums.com/threads/learning-social-rules-by-temple-grandin.13745

Hirota T, King BH. Autism spectrum disorder: a review. *JAMA.* 2023;329(2):157–168 PMID: 36625807 doi: 10.1001/jama.2022.23661

Love JR, Carr JE, Leblanc LA. Functional assessment of problem behavior in children with autism spectrum disorders: a summary of 32 outpatient cases. *J Autism Dev Disord.* 2009;39(2):363–372 PMID: 18704671 doi: 10.1007/s10803-008-0633-z

McGuire K, Fung LK, Hagopian L, et al. Irritability and problem behavior in autism spectrum disorder: a practice pathway for pediatric primary care. *Pediatrics.* 2016;137(suppl 2):S136–S148 PMID: 26908469 doi: 10.1542/peds.2015-2851L

Volkmar F, Siegel M, Woodbury-Smith M, King B, McCracken J, State M; American Academy of Child and Adolescent Psychiatry (AACAP) Committee on Quality Issues (CQI). Practice parameter for the assessment and treatment of children and adolescents with autism spectrum disorder. *J Am Acad Child Adolesc Psychiatry.* 2014;53(2):237–257 PMID: 24472258 doi: 10.1016/j.jaac.2013.10.013

CHAPTER 10

Diagnosing and Managing Co-Occurring Conditions

CASE VIGNETTE

Daniel is an 8-year-old verbal child with an average nonverbal intelligence quotient (IQ) who received a diagnosis of autism at 2 years of age. His parents make an appointment with their pediatric primary care clinician to discuss Daniel's difficulties staying seated and completing tasks in school. During his first years of elementary education, Daniel benefited from placement into a small noncategorical special education classroom, where he was felt to be meeting grade-level expectations. As a result, he was moved into a general education classroom for third grade. His teachers have never raised concerns for distractibility, hyperactivity, or inattention. His parents wonder if he would benefit from medication used for attention-deficit/hyperactivity disorder (ADHD).

Autism carries an increased risk for many co-occurring medical and psychiatric conditions that can negatively affect quality of life and long-term outcomes for children. The pediatric primary care clinician's role in screening and early identification of co-occurring conditions is essential to optimizing a child's developmental progress. Often the child and family will present concerns to the primary care clinician first, creating the opportunity for early treatment. The approach to identification and treatment of co-occurring conditions requires an individualized analysis of the child with an already complex and heterogeneous developmental disorder. The core features of autism can complicate the presentation of symptoms of evolving medical conditions, making their diagnosis more challenging. Many children and adolescents on the autism spectrum may be unable to express specific symptoms verbally, and the nonverbal presentations of externalizing behaviors, insomnia, or irritability are nonspecific. This chapter's case vignette opening illustrates the challenges involved in identifying coexisting conditions. The inattention that Daniel presents with in the case may be caused by challenges with impulse control and distraction, or it may reflect a core autism feature of restricted and repetitive behaviors that can interfere with the ability to focus on nonpreferred tasks. In the general education classroom, he is less likely to have the consistent level of support and accommodations to help him maintain his on-task behavior. Therefore, the shift into general education is likely to result in him having more difficulty attending to the tasks of the classroom.

Families may seek care for children who have nonspecific presentations, such as self-injurious behavior, aggression, or increasing perseverative behaviors, when the underlying issue is actually a secondary anxiety or a pain source, for example. As discussed in detail in Chapter 9, Autism and Behavioral Challenges: Why They Occur and How to Approach Them, it is imperative to understand the source of the behavior to determine if there is a specific trigger or if the behavior appears spontaneously and is indicative of a medical or psychiatric secondary phenomenon. The clinician may be faced with the question of whether increased head banging is an expression of frustration with a nonpreferred demand, is a response to a demand that is beyond that child's capacities, or is a reinforced behavior that allows escape and return to a preferred and soothing activity. In some cases, head banging might represent a secondary phenomenon unrelated to the demand, such as a source of pain or primary irritability. As another example, a child's food refusal might result from sensory aversions that are frequent features of autism, or it might be secondary to pain with eating caused by reflux disease, dental pain, or eosinophilic esophagitis. It is the role of the clinician to discern when a child's clinical presentation represents a coexisting secondary medical entity that is complicating autism in the presence of preexisting developmental challenges. A tool for monitoring symptoms in the context of autism and their commonly associated conditions is presented in Appendix A, Autism Monitoring Tool for the Pediatric Primary Care Clinician. This tool can be integrated into the electronic health record to screen for co-occurring conditions in children on the spectrum and monitor progress and treatment goals.

Many conditions seem to have a shared genetic heritability with autism and may be found in family members. Individuals who have a family member on the spectrum are at a 4-fold increased risk of having a diagnosis of ADHD and are at risk for a tic disorder, a seizure disorder, anxiety, social and pragmatic communication disorders, intellectual disability (ID), or schizophrenia.

Co-Occurring Neurological Conditions

Attention-Deficit/Hyperactivity Disorder

All subtypes of ADHD (inattentive, hyperactive-impulsive, and mixed subtypes) are far more common in children on the autism spectrum. Of the children diagnosed with ADHD alone, 1 in 8 will later receive a diagnosis of autism. Because datasets may represent different populations, reported ADHD prevalence among children on the spectrum varies.

Children on the spectrum evaluated by specialists tend to have more severe symptoms at presentation than those presenting in primary care. As a result, study samples chosen from neurology or psychiatry departments skew toward higher levels of co-occurring complexities, such as ADHD, when compared with autistic populations chosen from primary care settings. Reported prevalence rates of ADHD among autistic populations therefore vary from 40% to 70%. Coexisting autism and ADHD are associated with both increased needs around autism and increased incidence of other coexisting conditions such as anxiety and mood disorders. Children with more severe autism-associated challenges and co-occurring conditions warrant further evaluation and intensive treatment and monitoring given the risk for long-term negative effects on the child's well-being.

The *Diagnostic and Statistical Manual of Mental Disorders, Fifth Edition,* allows for the co-diagnosis of both entities, and although many of the clinical features and genetic risk factors overlap, ADHD and autism represent 2 distinct neurodevelopmental conditions of childhood, both of which may result in lifelong symptoms or difficulties, especially related to executive function skills. Although both ADHD and autism have clinical features related to executive functioning and social skills, the difficulties seen in each are specific and can be used to help differentiate one from the other. As a result of this distinction, they respond to different treatment approaches.

Executive function is a psychological term used to describe the skills required to allow an individual to stay on task and plan their thoughts and actions. These are commonly referred to as the "CEO" skills of the brain and they include the ability to inhibit responses, to shift one's focus, to plan, to use working memory, and to form concepts. Globally, these functions are more affected in the individual with ADHD. Those on the spectrum alone tend to have more selective difficulties with the demand for *cognitive flexibility* (the ability to quickly shift one's focus or perspective), whereas those with ADHD alone struggle more with *inhibition* (the ability to control a response), planning, and problem-solving. Differentiating executive functioning in individuals with ADHD versus those on the spectrum can be challenging and may require more formal psychological assessment.

Individuals with both ADHD and autism demonstrate difficulties in social functioning. In the context of ADHD, the social difficulty is most often related to the externalizing behaviors of impulsivity or hyperactivity (eg, intruding, blurting out responses), whereas those on the spectrum tend to have primary difficulties in their social skills. This includes their ability to interpret social cues and respond appropriately within social contexts.

It is necessary to distinguish when symptoms suggestive of ADHD are secondary to other entities such as anxiety, trauma, excessive media use, bullying, insomnia, or a lack of the supports needed by the child to be successful. Screening tools for ADHD such as the Vanderbilt Assessment Scales (https://publications.aap.org/pediatriccare/resources/17510/Vanderbilt-Assessment-Scales); the Swanson, Nolan and Pelham-IV (SNAP-IV); or the Conners Comprehensive Behavior Rating Scales (Conners CBRS) are used frequently by pediatric clinicians to aid in the diagnosis. Although these tools have not yet been adapted or standardized for children on the spectrum, they remain useful in better defining behavioral patterns and collecting information from observers. It is imperative that these tools be completed by adults in at least 2 settings (eg, home and school) to support the clinical assessment. Each child should be evaluated for the contributing features of autism and ADHD to help support the diagnosis. Psychological data looking at specific attentional functioning and executive function skills can be extremely helpful in evaluations of subtler and more complicated presentations, and patients who may have overlapping presentations may further benefit from a referral for full psychological testing to aid in diagnosis and treatment.

Response to pharmacologic intervention is not diagnostic of ADHD but may result in significant improvement in many children with or without a diagnosis of ADHD. The considerations for medication intervention are discussed in Chapter 13, Review of Pharmacotherapy and Complementary Interventions, but may be summarized by stating that children with coexisting autism and ADHD have less robust responses to medication in general and show less tolerance of standard titration doses. Therefore, children with combined ADHD and autism require a slow and careful prescribing pattern and close monitoring of symptoms. Although the supports needed in the autistic child and the child with ADHD are similar, autistic children tend to benefit from more global interventions and accommodations in addition to those needed for attentional regulation and executive function skills.

Other Neurological Features

Children on the autism spectrum are at increased risk for seizures, motor dysfunctions, stereotypical movement disorders, and insomnia. Some of these neurological features may be attributed to coexisting defined syndromes such as tuberous sclerosis complex or Rett syndrome (refer to Chapter 7, The Medical Evaluation of the Child Presumed or Confirmed to Be Autistic, for a full listing), but others represent the varied and heterogenous presentations of non-syndromic or idiopathic autism.

Seizures

Children, adolescents, and young adults on the autism spectrum are at significantly increased risk for seizures and epilepsy. Many will have abnormal or atypical findings on electroencephalography (EEG) without manifesting clinical features that require intervention. As a result, routine EEG is not recommended to screen asymptomatic individuals. Seizures have been reported to occur in 6% to 50% of individuals with an autism diagnosis and have a bimodal age distribution. There are 2 peaks for seizure presentation: the first in early childhood (ages 2–5 years) and the second in adolescence and adulthood. This bimodal pattern suggests different contributing etiologies, although this difference has not been elucidated. Those with an associated ID or genetic syndrome, and female children on the spectrum, are more likely to develop seizures and should be carefully monitored.

Any type of seizure is possible in children and adolescents on the spectrum, from absence seizures to generalized tonic-clonic presentations. Recognizing and interpreting seizure activity in a child on the spectrum can be challenging because the suspicious motor activity needs to be discriminated between a core feature of the repetitive behaviors of autism and that which is suggestive of seizures. Behaviors such as staring off, inattention, nighttime wakenings, eye deviation, and repetitive movements are often present in autistic individuals without seizures. Teachers or other adults who are not familiar with a child's history may report atypical or repetitive movements that have been present previously as an expression of their autism. Distinguishing a stereotypy, a tic, or a repetitive behavior of autism from that of a seizure disorder can be extremely challenging. It may be helpful for clinicians to teach adults who care for the child to differentiate movements of volition from those of seizures. Instructing adults to use a sudden gesture, sound, or touch to distract the child from a behavior may help distinguish between seizures and movements that can be redirected. Observing whether there is a change in mental status or consciousness can be a critical distinguishing feature. Requesting that parents record and share home videos of concerning motor activity may be helpful in assessing children presenting for possible seizure activity. These videos can help the pediatric primary care clinician discriminate between behaviors suggestive of seizure activity and those that are behavioral, secondary features of autism or of a different etiology. The motor activity observed in certain seizure phenomena may be characteristic and supportive of a specific diagnosis, such as infantile spasms or Lennox-Gastaut syndrome.

The children for whom significant concern for seizures is identified should be referred to a pediatric neurologist for diagnostic evaluation, including EEG, possible head imaging, and medication management if indicated. In most cases, the neurologist will order testing. Electroencephalography and correlation with video recordings may help support a diagnosis of epilepsy. In cases where a child is unable to tolerate a 24-hour video EEG telemetry and observation in the hospital, home ambulatory studies, although less optimal, may be a necessary first step before resorting to sedating a child for a study.

Motor Dysfunctions

Motor dysfunctions in autism are common and may manifest early, before a diagnosis can be made. These dysfunctions are varied and range from poor oral-motor skills, verbal apraxia (motor speech disorder), early head lag, poor motor imitation, or dysfunctions in skilled movements or praxis. *Praxis* refers to the planning and execution of motor tasks. This involves a series of actions that may seem routine but that may be problematic in a child with neurodevelopmental challenges. Examples include getting dressed, brushing one's teeth, or accessing playground equipment. Fine and gross motor skills may be affected. Gait abnormalities such as poor balance, toe walking, poor coordination, or postural abnormalities are often seen but are not specific to autism. Children on the autism spectrum may require additional instruction and practice when learning new motor skills and may benefit from physical therapy or the inclusion of motor skills in educational planning.

Some researchers and clinicians hypothesize that the motor dysfunctions of autism explain the lack of gesture use and inability to imitate motor actions. These dysfunctions in praxis can significantly affect the individual's everyday functioning and social experience. Although motor dysfunctions are often observed in autism to some degree, the extent of resulting difficulty may vary. It is important that children with suspected motor dysfunctions receive early referral for occupational therapy (OT) assessment and treatment integrated into their overall treatment planning.

Stereotypical and Repetitive Movements

The repetitive movements commonly seen in individuals on the autism spectrum may occur for a number of reasons: responses to stimuli, anxiety, self-stimulating, coping strategies, or self-soothing. They can vary from repetition of a single action (eg, closing doors, lining up objects) to rhythmic movements (eg, hand flapping, toe walking, finger flicking). These behaviors are predictable and often occur in specific settings, such as during times of stress or boredom or following a sensory stimulus. Addressing the underlying stress may result in improvement. The degree of effects resulting from these features of autism is variable. It is not necessary to treat to eradicate these behaviors, and an attempt to do so can result in significant stress for the autistic individual. If these behaviors are interfering with the child's ability to be successful, or they are disruptive to others, an attempt by a behavioral specialist or an OT to modify or redirect the child's behaviors may be indicated (eg, if the child is tapping a pencil on a table, perhaps tapping a soft object will be less audible to others). Educating peers about the cause and triggers of these behaviors can help them better understand the child and the behaviors they exhibit.

Insomnia

Sleep issues or insomnia is common in children and adolescents on the autism spectrum and can exacerbate the underlying challenges an autistic child experiences. Insomnia may be a primary or secondary disorder. The pediatric primary care clinician should be aware of this and screen the child at regular visits for sleep interruption and the need for intervention. Proactive counseling and preventive recommendations are helpful. Refer to Chapter 12, Insomnia: Identification and Interventions, for a thorough discussion of these topics.

Co-Occurring Gastrointestinal Symptoms

As many as 67% of children on the autism spectrum will experience gastrointestinal (GI) symptoms and restrictive eating patterns. There is no single GI disease that is specific to autism; therefore, each child needs to be evaluated individually. Gastrointestinal pathology in children on the spectrum may manifest with irritability, feeding difficulties, or escalation of autism features such as repetitive and stereotypical behaviors. Alternatively, GI disease in children on the spectrum may manifest with insomnia or an increase in externalizing or internalizing behaviors. Chapter 11, Gastrointestinal Symptoms and Feeding Challenges, reviews this topic in more detail.

Co-Occurring Behavioral Health Conditions

The majority of children on the autism spectrum (70%) will experience at least one associated behavioral health challenge, and 41% will experience 2 or more. The early identification and treatment of behavioral health concerns is particularly important within the context of autism. It is recommended that children on the spectrum undergo regular behavioral health screening, including screening for suicidality. Parents must be made aware of the increased risk for suicide in the autistic child. Recent analyses have reported that as many as 1 in 4 youth on the spectrum have had suicidal ideation and 1 in 10 have attempted suicide.

The most common manifesting behavioral health challenges for children on the spectrum, other than ADHD, are stress and anxiety (14%–50%) or depression (40%–80%). Risk factors for anxiety and depression during the teenage years include unmet support needs arising from higher cognitive capacity. Children with higher IQs are more likely to have less special education support and be in less restrictive educational environments. Many children may demonstrate strong developmental progress in their early years; however, as academic and social demands increase, they become more vulnerable to behavioral health challenges. Such challenges are not always readily identified, particularly when educational supports are limited and the child is less closely supervised. Heightened sensitivity to everyday sensory experiences and the escalating expectations of daily life may place them into more frequent states of hyperarousal.

Depression and anxiety in a child on the spectrum may manifest in a nonspecific manner, such as academic regression, externalizing behaviors, regressive behavior, decline in self-care, or exaggeration of autism features. The prototypical presentation seen in adults (change in appetite, sleep problems, or poor concentration) may not be obvious in children. All children in primary care should be screened as recommended by the American Academy of Pediatrics (AAP), and, additionally, when concerns are raised, with the use of standard screening tools for behavioral health concerns. There are many tools used in primary care such as the Pediatric Symptom Checklist-17 (PSC-17) for general screening. Level II screening is used for those where risk has already been identified, and one of the following tools is commonly used: the Screen for Child Anxiety Related Emotional Disorders (SCARED), the Patient Health Questionnaire-9 Modified for Adolescents (PHQ-A), or the Columbia DISC Depression Scale. The Ask Suicide-Screening Questions (ASQ) are used to screen for suicidality. (For a more thorough discussion of behavioral health screening tools, refer to the AAP "Screening Tools: Pediatric Mental Health Minute Series" page at www.aap.org/en/patient-care/mental-health-minute/screening-tools.)

Young people on the spectrum often have lower emotional self-awareness, which may limit the usefulness of self-report measures of behavioral health. For this reason, input from caregivers and other adults who know the child or adolescent well is essential. Standardized screening questionnaires should therefore be administered both to the autistic individual and to their caregivers.

Autism and Gender Identity and Sexuality

An increased prevalence of gender and sexuality diversity among individuals on the autism spectrum has been reported by clinicians and in research data. Gender and sexuality norms are ideas that determine how a person should look, behave, and identify according to their perceived gender as well as assigned sex at birth. The relationship between autism and gender variance is not well understood but is likely a combination of biological effects and the effect of the autistic individual's interpretation of societal expectations. Individuals on the spectrum are more likely to explore and express their gender identity and sexuality without adhering to societal norms. It is important for the clinician to consider the heterogeneity of expression when evaluating and caring for individuals on the spectrum and to recognize that gender dysphoria can manifest with significant concerns. It will be important, when possible, to screen or have an index of suspicion for gender variance in children and teens on the spectrum. Adolescents on the spectrum may struggle to identify and express gender dysphoria, gender identity, or sexual orientation. The questions asked when screening should be short and precise, such as "What gender are you?" Asking the questions while offering a safe opportunity for the teen to express their ideas about gender identity is helpful. The clinician may need to offer choices for responses (eg, cis male or female, trans male or female, and/or nonbinary/queer) and explanations of the terms being used. It may take time to clearly understand their experience. Families will benefit from an opportunity to discuss issues of gender identity and sexuality with their primary care clinician, who can model having this discussion without judgment. Ideally, these children and their parents should be referred to specialists in gender diversity who additionally have expertise in autism to complete assessments and consider when and if intervention is indicated. There are many resources available for parents to become more educated, such as those available through Autism Speaks (www.autismspeaks.org/lgbtq-identities).

CASE VIGNETTE: CONCLUSION

After careful consideration of Daniel's parents' concerns, the pediatric primary care clinician speaks with his teachers, reviews his individualized education program (IEP), and has his teachers and parents complete Vanderbilt Assessment Scales.

The scoring of the general education teacher questionnaire is highly suggestive of combined-type ADHD. The questionnaire responses reveal that Daniel demonstrates high levels of anxiety and self-consciousness about his behavior and that he always works very hard. His teacher reports that he is not successfully able to engage with peers during unstructured or organized activities. He seems anxious to try new things for fear of making mistakes. He struggles to maintain attention on tasks, avoids tasks requiring sustained attention, does not follow through when sustained effort and focus are required, is easily distracted and forgetful, becomes fidgety, moves about the room excessively, talks and blurts out responses, interrupts and intrudes into others' conversations, and loses things.

The special education teacher's responses on the Vanderbilt Assessment Scale do not support an ADHD diagnosis. She reports that in a small educational setting with behavioral supports, with instruction broken down into smaller demands, and with ample use of visual supports, Daniel is able to stay on task, follows through on instruction, appears relaxed, and performs productively in his academic tasks. The teacher describes his struggles with peer socialization and, in addition, his many restricted and repetitive tendencies and interests that seem to interfere with his ability to attend to demands and tasks.

Both parent questionnaire responses are subthreshold for an ADHD diagnosis as well, and Daniel's parents indicate that they have not observed any changes in his behavior in the home. He does well with routines that have been established, completes daily tasks, and follows through and stays organized for activities he is confident about and interested in. His parents note that his behavior at home is inconsistent and that they have had to work hard to motivate him in situations involving new learning or nonpreferred types of activities, especially those that involve language-based instruction. Further, they note that Daniel generally appears very anxious to know he is doing the right thing and wants to please others. He often expresses concern that his classmates do not like him. He has focused interests in the planets and some insects and, in general, talks at his parents rather than engages in conversational exchange and turn taking. Daniel has never been very interested in pretend and peer play.

On reviewing the IEP, the pediatric primary care clinician notices that Daniel is receiving special education support in reading and that otherwise he attends a general education class without accommodations or supports. The general education teacher's comments raise concern for inattention, distractibility, and hyperactivity, but the primary concerns focus on Daniel's restricted and repetitive interests, need for structure and support for his on-task behavior, and anxiety. In their responses, his teachers note that Daniel works slowly, struggles to transition and try new tasks, and insists on making his work

Continued on next page

"perfect" before handing it in. When the work is interesting to him, he is able to sustain his focus. His psychological testing demonstrates that he has the cognitive, linguistic, and problem-solving skills to successfully participate in grade-level curricula but processes information and language slowly and has executive function challenges. Additionally, his focused and atypical interests are described, as well as a struggle with showing reciprocal social engagement and fitting in with his peer group.

The primary care clinician shares the conclusions with Daniel's parents: Daniel requires more support in the general education classroom before any consideration of a medical treatment should be made. The IEP team meets again to review accommodations and supports that would benefit Daniel, with the goal of lessening his anxiety and increasing his ability to stay on task and complete his work. The team assembles accommodations, a positive behavior plan, preparation for transition, plans to include his preferred interests in lessons, and visual supports that break down instruction into small segments.

Daniel makes tremendous improvements during the following semester; both his anxiety and his work improve. Despite this progress, the primary care clinician initiates a medication trial after Daniel's general education teacher continues to observe inattention, distractibility, and hyperactivity that interfere with his ability to stay on task. The primary care clinician determines that ADHD is interfering with Daniel's ability to progress in a less restrictive environment. In situations where more special education support is not available, initiating a medication trial is reasonable. Daniel is prescribed a very low dose of a stimulant, and a 2-week follow-up appointment is scheduled to titrate his dose as tolerated.

The improvement over the course of the academic year is remarkably positive. Daniel meets with the primary care clinician on a regular basis, and his parents share data from his school reports. Daniel's progress is demonstrated in his academic performance across the board and confirmed by his teachers' responses on follow-up Vanderbilt Assessment Scale questionnaires. Daniel's pride in his accomplishments is evident to his teachers, his parents, and the primary care clinician, and there is a clear decrease in his anxiety. The IEP team explains that further monitoring of Daniel's social skills and his anxiety is imperative and suggests consideration of his placement into a social skills group to work on pragmatic social skills and flexibility.

This case vignette exemplifies how a careful collection of data obtained from direct testing as well as responses from professionals and parents can enable the pediatric primary care clinician to understand the child's level of functioning, challenges, and needs for support. Understanding the nature of the educational services and accommodations was important for determining next steps. (The special education process and how it applies to the primary care clinician is discussed in more detail in Chapter 14, Working With Special Education Services: A Primer.) The data from the psychoeducational testing supported a logical sequence of operationalizing interventions with an emphasis on educational interventions first, before making a diagnosis of ADHD and turning to a medication trial. The cumulative effect of educational supports and a medication trial helped support Daniel's successes with lessened expression of stress and anxiety. In this case, the primary barrier to Daniel's progress was related to his autism, but struggles with attentional regulation and distractibility were interfering with his ability to progress in a general education environment. Further concern for anxiety and delayed social skills identified new areas to address. This case is an example of how the pediatric primary care clinician's involvement can result in benefits to the child's treatment plan and performance. Discussions with Daniel's parents broadened their understanding of his needs and identified ways they could support him in the home, and the primary care clinician was able to collaborate with the school to support Daniel's progress.

The common occurrence of somatic as well as behavioral health disorders in children on the autism spectrum can lead to the exacerbation of developmental challenges and physical distress. These co-occurring conditions contribute to the heterogeneity of the clinical presentations of autism and the complexity of autism care. This heterogeneity requires a systematic approach for monitoring progress and making therapeutic recommendations. Differentiating when autism has a co-occurring secondary physiological or behavioral entity is imperative and will affect treatment recommendations.

Clinical Pearls

- Autism carries an increased risk for many medical and psychiatric conditions that can negatively affect quality of life and long-term outcomes.
- The pediatric primary care clinician's role in screening and early identification of co-occurring conditions is essential to a child's developmental course.
- Often the child and family will present concerns to the primary care clinician first, creating the opportunity for early assessment and treatment.
- All subtypes of ADHD (inattentive, hyperactive-impulsive, and mixed subtypes) are far more common in children on the autism spectrum.
- Children on the spectrum are at increased risk for seizures, motor dysfunctions, stereotypical movement, and sleep disorders.
- The majority of children on the spectrum (70%) will have at least one associated behavioral health challenge, and 41% will have 2 or more.
- As many as 67% of children on the spectrum will experience GI symptoms.

References

Antshel KM, Russo N. Autism spectrum disorders and ADHD: overlapping phenomenology, diagnostic issues, and treatment considerations. *Curr Psychiatry Rep.* 2019;21(5):34 PMID: 30903299 doi: 10.1007/s11920-019-1020-5

Bougeard C, Picarel-Blanchot F, Schmid R, Campbell R, Buitelaar J. Prevalence of autism spectrum disorder and co-morbidities in children and adolescents: a systematic literature review. *Front Psychiatry.* 2021;12:744709 PMID: 34777048 doi: 10.3389/fpsyt.2021.744709

Carroll LS, Owen MJ. Genetic overlap between autism, schizophrenia and bipolar disorder. *Genome Med.* 2009;1(10):102 PMID: 19886976 doi: 10.1186/gm102

Huggins CF, Donnan G, Cameron IM, Williams JH. Emotional self-awareness in autism: a meta-analysis of group differences and developmental effects. *Autism.* 2021;25(2):307–321 PMID: 33153301 doi: 10.1177/1362361320964306

Mansour R, Dovi AT, Lane DM, Loveland KA, Pearson DA. ADHD severity as it relates to comorbid psychiatric symptomatology in children with autism spectrum disorders (ASD). *Res Dev Disabil.* 2017;60:52–64 PMID: 27889487 doi: 10.1016/j.ridd.2016.11.009

Maski KP, Jeste SS, Spence SJ. Common neurological co-morbidities in autism spectrum disorders. *Curr Opin Pediatr.* 2011;23(6):609–615 PMID: 21970828 doi: 10.1097/MOP.0b013e32834c9282

O'Halloran L, Coey P, Wilson C. Suicidality in autistic youth: a systematic review and meta-analysis. *Clin Psychol Rev.* 2022;93:102144 PMID: 35290800 doi: 10.1016/j.cpr.2022.102144

Simonoff E, Pickles A, Charman T, Chandler S, Loucas T, Baird G. Psychiatric disorders in children with autism spectrum disorders: prevalence, comorbidity, and associated factors in a population-derived sample. *J Am Acad Child Adolesc Psychiatry.* 2008;47(8):921–929 PMID: 18645422 doi: 10.1097/CHI.0b013e318179964f

Strang JF, Meagher H, Kenworthy L, et al. Initial clinical guidelines for co-occurring autism spectrum disorder and gender dysphoria or incongruence in adolescents. *J Clin Child Adolesc Psychol.* 2018;47(1):105–115 PMID: 27775428 doi: 10.1080/15374416.2016.1228462

CHAPTER 11

Gastrointestinal Symptoms and Feeding Challenges

CASE VIGNETTE

The office receives a phone call from a parent expressing concern about their 10-year-old child Amir, who is well-known to the practice. Amir received a diagnosis of autism in the preschool years and has very limited communication skills. He attends school in a self-contained autism-centered classroom. For years, Amir's pediatric primary care clinician has been working with his family to support healthy eating patterns. Amir has a very restrictive diet, eating frozen pancakes from one specific brand, plain potato chips, sweetened strawberry yogurt, and vanilla milkshakes from a specific fast-food chain. Amir's parent reaches out today because Amir has increasingly developed a low frustration tolerance and has started biting himself and banging his head when upset. Amir's teachers and school staff cannot find any specific patterns or triggers for this behavior, and they have shared with Amir's parents that the behavior is pervasive and interferes with his learning and engagement.

Because of the common occurrence of gastrointestinal (GI) symptoms in children on the autism spectrum and the significance they have on a child's quality of life, knowledge of the effects of these symptoms is important for clinicians caring for children on the spectrum. Autistic individuals with GI involvement experience poorer long-term quality of life than those without GI issues. Children on the spectrum therefore require regular surveillance and a high index of suspicion for coexisting GI disease with the knowledge that their presenting symptoms may be nonspecific. The early identification of GI diagnoses will prevent secondary sequelae and result in more rapid resolution of symptoms that would otherwise persist.

Gastrointestinal symptoms and food selectivity may co-occur in up to 75% of children on the spectrum, although the reported prevalence varies. Children on the spectrum who have GI involvement are likely to experience abdominal pain, constipation, diarrhea, gastroesophageal reflux disease (GERD), pain with stooling, and/or food selectivity. Symptoms vary and there is no one specific GI etiology or recommendation for treatment.

Because of communication challenges, children on the spectrum may struggle to localize the source of their discomfort, which can complicate the diagnostic process. Gastrointestinal involvement, therefore, may manifest as a behavioral concern, and adults caring for the child may make assumptions and interpret patterns of irritability and/or disruptive behavior without attending to the possibility of underlying organic causes. Rather than report specific GI symptoms, autistic children with GI symptoms may present with increases in anxiety, externalizing behavior, somatic concerns, sleep irregularities, and reactivity to sensory stimuli. These types of presentations might appear as increases in tics, throat clearing, whining, crying, echoing statements about their stomach, agitation, repetitive behaviors, aggression, self-injurious behavior, or task avoidance.

This chapter's case vignette opening illustrates a common presentation for a child on the spectrum who may or may not have underlying GI pathology. Evaluating children with GI symptoms requires a differential diagnostic approach and careful review of the history. The first step of this evaluation involves a careful history of the child's sleep, diet, and toileting, as well as a review of behavior and other potential contributors (**Box 11.1**). In addition, a thorough medical review looking for other sources of pain (eg, dental concerns, ear infection, headache) or irritation (eg, pruritus, eczema) is indicated. A list of findings and prioritized treatment plans should be developed and implemented sequentially. Parent education and resource sharing are a part of providing a medical home for children. A representative sampling of resources for parents is listed at the end of this chapter.

The child may exhibit subtle expressions of their autism that can mimic or complicate symptoms of co-occurring processes. Understanding the chronology of the GI symptoms is important. For example, children on the spectrum are at risk for food selectivity given the common presence of sensory or textural preferences with eating. Many children will insist on a limited repertoire that has a similar appearance, color, texture, and/or smell. These children may be slow to incorporate new foods into their diet and require many presentations with increasing exposures. These background chronic issues might cloud the assessments of new and evolving GI pathology when more acute symptoms manifest. Commonly seen GI symptoms include abdominal pain, constipation, diarrhea, and feeding challenges. Individuals on the spectrum may also have GI disease that requires evaluation, such as celiac disease, eosinophilic esophagitis, GERD, or food allergies. Likewise, chronic issues can be exacerbated by new psychosocial stressors, anxiety or depression, or sources of discomfort. A review of behavioral management in the home and in

BOX 11.1 History Questionnaire for the Autistic Child With Gastrointestinal Symptoms

Circle or write the parent's response as indicated.

1. Sleep history				
Bedtime resistance:	Yes	No		
Nighttime wakening:	Yes	No		
Amount of sleep per night on average:				
2. Stooling habits				
Frequency:	More than twice daily			
	Daily			
	Every other day			
	Less than 3 times per week			
Consistency:	Hard	Small pellets	Normal	
	Soft	Runny	No form	
Pain:	Yes	No		
3. Toilet training history				
Resists, withholds:	Yes	No		
Fecal soiling:	Yes	No		
Prior treatment of GI symptoms:				
4. Other GI symptoms				
Abdominal pain:	Yes	No		
Vomiting:	Yes	No		
5. Feeding history				
Schedule for meals and snack:	Regular	Erratic		
Sits at table:	Yes	No		
Snacks often:	Yes	No		
Grazes as desired:	Yes	No		
Feeds self:	Yes	No		
Fed by parent:	Yes	No		
Parent uses distraction or force:	Yes	No		
Fed while sleeping:	Yes	No		
6. Diet				
Eats healthy variety:	Yes	No		
Limited repertoire:	Yes	No		
If yes, please explain:				
Highly selective:	Yes	No		
Textural preferences:	Yes	No		
Drinks (oz):	Milk	Juice	Soda	Other
7. Psychosocial history				
Stress:	Yes	No		
Loss:	Yes	No		
Trauma:	Yes	No		
Financial/food insecurity:	Yes	No		

Abbreviation: GI, gastrointestinal.

therapeutic environments is required to ensure that there is no secondary gain from the child's behavior that is contributing to the behavioral manifestations. It may be helpful to request a professional behavioral assessment to better understand the function of a manifesting behavior as its etiology is being considered.

Constipation

The most common GI symptom for children on the autism spectrum is constipation (with or without encopresis). The pediatric primary care clinician can provide care for most children on the spectrum who present with constipation in the same way as they would for any child with these symptoms. The treatments and management strategies that are used for all children with constipation can result in significant relief for those on the spectrum. A meta-analysis was performed and an algorithm created to guide the management of constipation in children, providing the pediatric primary care clinician and the specialist with a tiered approach (**Figure 11.1**).

When a child presents with a history of fewer than 3 bowel movements per week, the diagnosis of constipation is made. The clinician will perform a physical examination and review the relevant medical history. A careful analysis of causality should include assessment for contributing medical causes as reviewed in **Box 11.2**. Medical causes such as celiac disease, hypothyroidism, and food intolerance should be considered in the differential diagnosis. Children on the spectrum may have a limited dietary repertoire resulting in limited fiber and fluid intake and an altered gut microbiome. Children on the spectrum may spend less time in physical exercise and more time in sedentary activities, both of which can further contribute to struggles with constipation. Those with chronic constipation and encopresis can progress such that fecal withholding and toileting refusal develop as secondary avoidance of the pain associated with rectal emptying. These children require behavioral and/or psychological counseling, a behavioral treatment program, and medical management.

Intervention is recommended in the child with fewer than 3 bowel movements per week as indicated in **Box 11.3**. The presence of the following "red flag" symptoms

BOX 11.2 Causes of Constipation in Children and Adolescents on the Autism Spectrum

1. Medical conditions: celiac disease, hypothyroidism, or low muscle tone
2. Dietary deficiencies: may arise from decreased amounts of fruits and vegetables, inadequate fiber, poor fluid intake, or excessive milk intake in lieu of a balanced diet
3. Fecal withholding: may occur secondary to toilet training, sensory issues around using the toilet, fear from associated pain, lack of motivation to use the toilet, resistance to leaving a preferred activity to use the toilet, or a change in routine
4. Additional factors: lack of exercise, illness

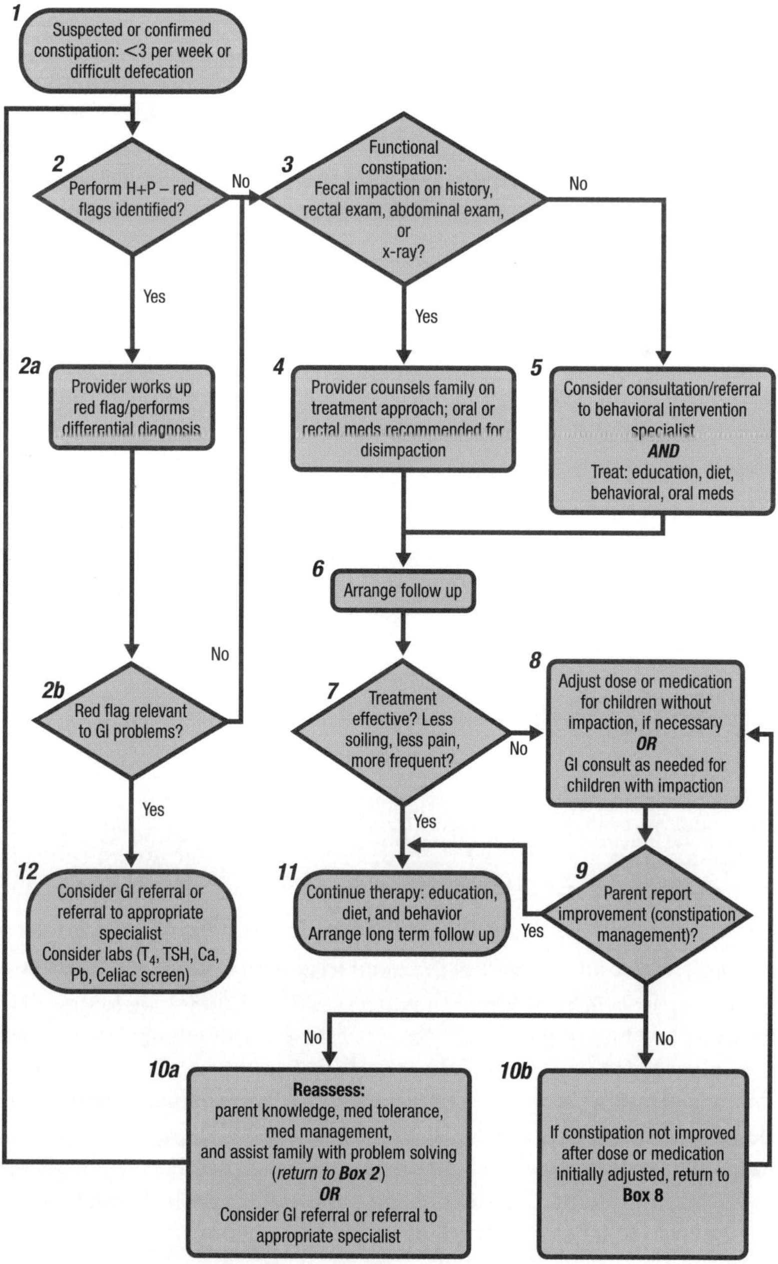

Figure 11.1. Algorithm for Treatment of Constipation in Children

Ca indicates calcium; exam, examination; GI, gastrointestinal; H+P, history and physical examination; lab, laboratory test; med, medication; Pb, lead; T_4, thyroxine; and TSH, thyroid-stimulating hormone.

Adapted from Furuta GT, Williams K, Kooros K, et al. Management of constipation in children and adolescents with autism spectrum disorders. *Pediatrics.* 2012;130(suppl 2):S98–S105.

BOX 11.3 When to Initiate Treatment of Constipation

1. Fewer than 3 bowel movements per week, possibly associated with one or more of the following symptoms: painful stooling, change in caliber of stool, abdominal pain, fecal soiling, change in appetite
2. "Red flag" symptoms indicating a need for referral: pain, poor weight gain, abdominal distention, nausea, vomiting, concern for tethered cord

indicates the need for either a referral to an appropriate specialist or the ordering of laboratory tests to pursue a medical etiology: fever, abdominal distension, anorexia, nausea, vomiting, poor weight gain or weight loss, lack of lumbosacral curve, presence of pilonidal dimple, or abnormal findings on lower extremity neurological examination.

Medical management using polyethylene glycol (PEG) as a first-line treatment of both constipation and impaction can be successful in providing initial relief (**Box 11.4**). If the determination is made that the child is impacted and having fecal soiling as a result, the disimpaction regimen will be used before moving to a maintenance regimen.

Some children, especially those with preexisting sensory aversions, may struggle to ingest oral medications, and alternatives may be necessary. PEG has little taste and is generally well tolerated, but if oral medications or an alternative (as listed in **Box 11.4**) are refused, the use of enemas, senna syrup, or bisacodyl suppositories is recommended. Some children may have discomfort with medication treatment; therefore, a slower titration may be needed. To sustain regular stooling and prevent relapse, it is essential to use maintenance medication while referring for or initiating appropriate dietary and nonmedical behavioral therapies.

Constipation may occur in children in whom fecal withholding and toileting avoidance have developed. Withholding might occur secondary to pain experienced with rectal emptying after an episode of rectal irritation or transient constipation. In other situations, withholding may be caused by toileting avoidance related to toilet training and sensory vulnerabilities. These children will benefit from behavioral therapy with occupational therapists (OTs), psychotherapists, or behavioral therapists experienced with toileting refusal. Before behavioral therapy is initiated, it is important that the constipation is well controlled with medication and that the child is no longer experiencing painful stooling.

The behavioral treatment plan for fecal withholding and/or toileting avoidance includes having the child sit on the toilet after meals, to take advantage of the gastrocolic reflex. It is important to choose a toilet option that is comfortable for the child and allows their feet to rest on a surface. Some children may prefer a small training toilet on the floor, and others may prefer a stable seat placed onto the toilet.

BOX 11.4 Treatment of Constipation and Impaction

1. **Medication**
   Disimpaction: 1 to 1.5 g/kg/day of PEG 3350 for 3 days followed by maintenance doses
   Maintenance doses:
   - PEG: 0.5 to 1 g/kg/day

   or
   - Lactulose: 1 to 3 mL/kg/day

   or
   - Milk of magnesia: 1 to 3 mL/kg/day

   Alternative medications for maintenance:
   - Lactulose: 1 to 3 mL/kg/day, in divided doses
   - Senna: ½ to 1 square daily for 3 days (Use with caution, as it may cause increased cramping.)
2. **Increase in regular exercise:** Exercise has been demonstrated to relieve constipation. Clinicians should encourage families to find activities that the child finds motivating and that respect the child's sensory needs. Making these activities easily available will lead to more success. Some families will create a space in their house for exercise. If a parent requests additional ideas or support, the clinician can refer the child for occupational therapy or refer the family to the resource *The Out-of-Sync Child Has Fun: Activities for Kids with Sensory Processing Disorder,* Revised Edition, by Carol Stock Kranowitz.
3. **Bowel habit training:** Clinicians can offer the following guidance to parents to support the establishment of healthy bowel habits:
   - Introduce a regular time to sit on the toilet. Observe when the child typically has a bowel movement and use this time as a starting point for regular toilet time.
   - Increase the amount of time spent on the toilet to no more than 5 to 10 minutes to optimize success and avoid resistance.
   - Use reinforcers for following instructions. Consider a positive reinforcement system through which the child obtains an extrinsic reward for completing a specified routine. A point system or a tangible reward can be used based on the child's developmental abilities.
   - Use a visual schedule for toileting and have pictures of each step involved. (Many such tools are available online or through a therapist.)
4. **Sensory considerations:** Some children struggle with the transition from a diaper and associated privacy to the use of a toilet. Parents can experiment with what types of toilet the child is most comfortable with so their feet are resting on a surface and they feel secure, comfortable, and stable. Some restroom environments may be aversive to some children because of the presence of other people, hand driers, or automatic flushers. These types of potentially aversive stimuli should be considered along with possible accommodations in a quieter restroom. Many schools have alternatives available, such as single-use bathrooms.
5. **Feeding therapy:** Clinicians may refer children with a limited dietary repertoire to a feeding therapist (refer to the Feeding Challenges section later in this chapter) to enhance dietary intake of fiber, fluids, and a healthy variety of wholesome foods.

Abbreviation: PEG, polyethylene glycol.

The parent can help the child practice the Valsalva maneuver by gently pressing on the child's abdomen with a pillow or teaching the child to blow at a pinwheel or rapidly exhale. When a child feels anxious or avoidant, a behavioral program can also help them transition to the use of the toilet with positive reinforcement for each step achieved. This might involve allowing them to request a diaper for bowel movements first and then gradually encouraging them to stand progressively closer to the toilet. At first, the child might attempt to leave the room, but gradually they should be able to tolerate being guided to move closer to the bathroom, to move into the bathroom, and, eventually, to have the bowel movement while standing next to the toilet. The next step would be learning to sit on the toilet while wearing a diaper. If the parent is unable to move toward removing the diaper, they may try placing a slit in the diaper to allow the bowel movement to fall into the toilet. The parent then gradually cuts back the material on the diaper until the child is able to sit and empty without the diaper.

Children on the spectrum who have a history of chronic selective eating are likely to experience persistent constipation resulting from poor fiber and fluid intake and can benefit from nutritional and feeding therapy as the constipation is treated.

The child's response to treatment requires ongoing supervision by the pediatric primary care clinician to avoid the tendency for the child to develop increased withholding, impaction, and further discomfort. The primary care clinician should supervise medical management and ensure that the child is maintaining regular stooling without discomfort, while behavioral intervention should address maintenance of healthy habits and the prevention of relapse. A maintenance phase using both medication and behavioral intervention is likely to be needed for months to years.

Feeding Challenges

The feeding challenges seen with children on the autism spectrum may be more common and extreme than those seen with typically developing children. Children on the spectrum may refuse to try new foods, require more repeated exposures of new foods before they will willingly eat them, have specific sensory needs for the foods they will tolerate, and have a restrictive set of rituals around eating. All these tendencies may persist into adulthood and have significant effects and may present challenges to the family. The primary care clinician is positioned to identify these challenges at an early age and intervene before they negatively affect the child's well-being. Feeding challenges tend not to spontaneously resolve on their own and, in fact, may worsen over time with resultant nutritional deficiencies and emotional distress for the child and their caregivers.

Sensory aversions and food selectivity are the most common reasons for feeding challenges. The child may refuse certain food groups, textures, smells, and visual presentations. Most children on the spectrum who have feeding challenges take in adequate calories and have adequate growth, but their challenges eventually become a risk factor for iron deficiency anemia; vitamin D, calcium, zinc, or other micronutrient deficiencies; and obesity later in life.

It is not unusual for autistic children to exhibit types of selective eating that may include a preference for simple carbohydrates; an aversion to fruits and vegetables; restrictiveness about food presentation, temperature, or texture; and not allowing foods to touch or be mixed together. The child may eat only a certain brand of food, and their diet may become progressively more restrictive over time. These restrictive patterns of eating can progress from concerning to dangerous if one of the preferred-brand foods has a change in formulation or is no longer commercially available. In these circumstances, a child with restrictive intake may refuse to eat a replacement food.

Children on the spectrum may be averse to touching or smelling food or watching another person eat a particular food. These types of sensory aversions can result in such extreme hyper-selectivity that the child meets the criteria for avoidant/restrictive food intake disorder (ARFID), because of the extent of their limited intake.

The clinician should evaluate for possible factors contributing to food aversions by first looking for red flags, or warning signs, and then looking for underlying medical causes that may inform the treatment plan. Contributing factors to feeding challenges are summarized in **Box 11.5**. The presence of associated pain or vomiting with eating, poor growth, lethargy, abdominal pain or masses, irritability, constipation, coughing, or choking should trigger a medical evaluation for causation. A careful history should be elicited and, if possible, an observation of a feeding interaction should be made either in person or via video. The pediatric primary care clinician may initiate this assessment, but in most cases, the child should be referred to a pediatric gastroenterologist and a feeding specialist.

BOX 11.5 Factors Contributing to Feeding Challenges

- Medical causes and related symptoms
  - Gastroesophageal reflux disease with possible food allergy/eosinophilic esophagitis: pain with feeding, recurrent vomiting, growth failure, pallor, lethargy, or eczema
  - Constipation: abdominal pain, self-injurious behavior, externalizing behaviors
  - Dysphagia: coughing, choking, or drooling
- Food avoidance or aversion: aversions to eating caused by associated experiences; specific foods, textures, or smells; or, in the extreme situation with more global restrictions, avoidant/restrictive food intake disorder
- Behavioral contributors: inability to sit at the table, resistant behavior, throwing, aversive parenting
- Parent-child interactions during feeding: coercive practices, use of distraction (eg, video) or use of bottle-feeding while the child is asleep

The child with feeding challenges will likely benefit from working with a feeding therapist with behavioral expertise for an assessment of triggers and reinforcers of the feeding refusals. An observation may determine which antecedent events might trigger the refusal (eg, specific foods, other conditions) or might identify a secondary gain achieved from the behavior. This observation should seek to evaluate what the dynamics of the parent-child interaction are and how these dynamics may contribute to the behaviors being addressed.

The child with food aversions will likely require regular feeding therapy in addition to behavioral supports. The pediatric primary care clinician can offer suggestions that may result in immediate significant improvement while the child is waiting to obtain feeding therapy. These recommendations might include providing a meal schedule while minimizing snacking, offering fluids only after the meal, and/or using positive reinforcers for sitting at the table for meals. **Box 11.6** provides a thorough list of suggested feeding strategies that clinicians can review and share with parents.

BOX 11.6 Feeding Strategies for Parents and Caregivers

- **Use positive incentives.** Attend to desired behaviors with verbal acknowledgement: "I like the way you are sitting" or "Thank you for trying a new food." Make eye contact, smile, and engage when the child is demonstrating the readiness behaviors that are desired. Praise the child's readiness behaviors while avoiding praise related to the amount of food the child eats.
- **Do not reinforce negative behaviors.** Avoid attending to undesirable behaviors, such as refusals, aggression, tantrums, or throwing. Observe if the child's behavior results in their gaining access to what they prefer (getting down from the table, eating in front of a screen, getting only preferred foods, or gaining access to objects they want). Avoid comments that could lead to power struggles over the meal (eg, commenting on what or how much the child has eaten).
- **Make mealtimes relaxed.** Support a pleasant mealtime experience and refrain from commenting on what the child eats. Avoid conflict, remove distracters, and avoid engaging in tasks away from the table (eg, answering the phone, doing dishes). Do not clean the child or the area, scold them, or make demands of them during the meal.
- **Make the child comfortable.** Have the child sit at the table when rested and in a happy mood. Use a comfortable and supportive chair where the child's feet rest on a surface. Children with low muscle tone may benefit from occupational therapy input on the use of supportive equipment for feeding.
- **Allow the child some control.** Offer choices, provide one spoon for the child and another for the parent, and allow the child to self-feed as much as possible. Set goals together and make a feeding schedule that the child can see.
- **Provide consistency.** Aim to provide 3 meals and 2 snacks per day. Allow the child to eat only when seated at the table.

BOX 11.6 *(continued)*

- **Avoid continual snacking.** Allow the child to eat only at scheduled meal and snack times and have water only in between these designated times.
- **Limit mealtimes.** Set a realistic expectation for sitting at the table to minimize power struggles and maximize success: meal duration should be limited to a maximum of 20 minutes.
- **Do not use distractions to encourage success.** Distractions, such as screens and devices, should not be used while eating. To encourage the child to sit at the table, try providing fun activities while the child is seated there before a meal. Alternatively, allow the child to take a break from eating to reinforce their behavior with a fun activity at the table before resuming eating. Distractions during eating should be avoided, as they do not encourage the child's participation in the meal.
- **Involve the child in meal planning and other meal-related activities.** Include the child in food selections and meal preparations. For older children and for those with the cognitive capacity to understand, discuss the effects of healthy eating on the body and growth and allow them to learn about food groups while involving them in recipe and food selection, planning, shopping, and preparation.
- **Expose the child to sensory experiences with food.** When a new food is introduced, allow the child to smell or touch the food; then, gradually increase their exposure to the food by bringing the food to their mouth, having them kiss or lick the food, and, eventually, having them take a bite. The child's involvement in meal preparation can likewise expose them to the sensory experiences needed to build tolerance to new foods.
- **Build on the foods the child likes.** Observe which foods the child prefers and then add new similar foods gradually and in small amounts. Start by using a new brand, flavor, or preparation of a preferred food, or a new food that has a similar texture to a preferred food. To meet nutritional goals, the nonpreferred foods may be masked by the foods the child prefers. For example, if the child likes milk, use milk to make a smoothie with fruit, a vegetable, or peanut butter. If the child likes pancakes, add extra eggs, cream, pureed fruits, or vegetables to the batter to augment the calories and the nutritional value. The goal of making each bite of food calorically and nutritionally dense is helpful in meeting a child's nutritional needs. When adding a new food, use very small amounts at first and gradually increase the additions.
- **Offer 1 to 2 foods the child likes along with 1 new food.** Make serving sizes small and encourage repeated and gradually increased exposure. Use the same food, repeatedly, until the food is accepted.
- **Offer solids before liquids.** Offering solids first helps avoid a feeding challenge in which the child is relying solely on liquids and becoming full by drinking. If the child will take only fluids, find ways to enhance them nutritionally by concentrating formula; adding nut butters, fruits, powdered milk, or yogurt; or using nutritional supplement drinks, such as PediaSure, or other prescribed nutritional supplements.
- **Have realistic expectations.** Anticipate periods of transition and do not expect a child to eat a full serving of a food on the first exposure. It may take weeks for a child to accept a new food.
- **Introduce a multivitamin with zinc after a careful dietary history is elicited.**

In the case of ARFID, specific strategies, in addition to behavioral practices, can be helpful when attempting to introduce new foods. These practices are beyond the scope of a primary care–directed intervention and involve food chaining. They are discussed in more detail in the parent resources referenced at the end of this chapter and are introduced by experienced feeding therapists. They involve building on the child's preferences and making small changes when choosing a new food to introduce. While waiting for the child to be accepted to a feeding therapy program, the pediatric primary clinician might make the recommendations listed in **Box 11.6**.

Food Allergies and Elimination Diets

The link between immune and autoimmune processes and autism has been described in the research literature. The data demonstrate that if there is a family history of autoimmune disease, there will be an increased likelihood of a family member being on the autism spectrum. A recent survey of 200,000 parents of children who received an autism diagnosis showed a connection between autism and parent-reported food allergies. The study revealed that 11.25% of children on the spectrum were reported by parents to have food allergies, compared to 4.25% of typically developing children. This association between reported food allergies and autism was especially prevalent among children with increased needs around autism.

An increased association of respiratory and skin allergies has also been reported among children on the spectrum. There are no data to support specific types of associated allergies or a causal relationship with autism, but it is important for the pediatric primary care clinician to be alert to these possible contributors to a child's irritability and GI symptoms.

The data on links between autism and specific food allergies such as gluten and casein allergies have been inconclusive. This is a research area that is methodologically difficult to study in a blinded and controlled manner. Many lay groups make strong recommendations about the efficacy of elimination diets, so parents may bring these suggestions to the pediatric primary care clinician for discussion or will pursue elimination diets independently. The research results are varied and have drawn inconsistent conclusions. The one study by Elder that was blinded and controlled showed no demonstrable or statistically significant difference in symptoms between autistic children prescribed a gluten-free and casein-free (GFCF) diet and those maintaining a standard diet. Interestingly, the parents in the study were very invested in the elimination diet and were reluctant to reintroduce these foods even after the negative results were shared. A large recent meta-analysis showed no consistent or demonstrable beneficial association between a GFCF diet and symptoms in autistic children. There is, therefore, no data to support the recommendation of a GFCF diet for all children on the spectrum despite parents often being invested in its use.

The available research data do not support a universal approach to food allergies in the context of autism. When there are concerns for persistent food refusal, bowel irregularities, irritability, the presence of atopic disease, or parental reports of associations between the ingestion of certain foods and concerning symptoms, food allergies should be considered and either the introduction of elimination diets or a referral to an allergist for testing is recommended. Nutritional guidance is also recommended to ensure adequate nutritional variety and to avoid the tendency to progressively narrow food choices.

Obesity and Associated Concerns

Children on the autism spectrum are known to have a higher predisposition for excessive weight gain and subsequent obesity compared with their non-autistic peers. Excessive weight gain and overweight (>85th percentile body mass index [BMI]) or obesity (>95th percentile BMI) puts a child at risk for lifelong issues that include diabetes, heart disease, and insulin resistance and can compound risk factors known to exist with autism. It is likely that the sensory-driven selective eating patterns, high intake of processed foods, and more sedentary lifestyle often seen in those on the spectrum increase the child's risk for obesity. Both the prevalence of sleep disorders and the frequent use of antipsychotic medications are likely to contribute to obesity. Additionally, there is evidence for leptin resistance possibly leading to an interference with the healthy regulation of appetite and energy expenditure in those on the spectrum. There is some evidence for decreased gut microbiome diversity in those on the spectrum, although the findings are inconsistent. These changes are hypothesized to lead to the increased production of inflammatory cytokines possibly implicated in the development of autism. It is important that the primary care clinician evaluate each child's risk factors for excessive weight gain, educate families, and individualize the treatment plan accordingly. This assessment and treatment plan should focus on a dietary history and treatment that will result in a varied diet rich in whole foods. Early intervention is essential to achieve this goal.

CASE VIGNETTE: CONCLUSION

When Amir returns for a pediatric visit, his parents share that his very selective diet has become more limited, as the brands of strawberry yogurt and the milkshake he used to eat are no longer available. He will not take any other brands as replacements and his diet is now short of protein and overall nutritional content. Amir's parents and educators are concerned about his poor nutrition. Mealtimes have become increasingly difficult, and Amir's parents and teachers find that he is adamant in his refusals and more irritable overall.

Continued on next page

On further history, the clinician learns that Amir avoids sitting on the toilet, has frequent fecal smearing, and is stooling less than 3 times per week. Amir's teachers report that his irritability is interfering with his attention to learning and that he has been more disruptive in the classroom, causing them to release him to an aide to walk the halls. On further investigation, Amir's teacher had introduced a new educational goal requiring him to produce all handwritten work rather than to rely on the computer to type his responses. Amir is not meeting this goal, despite his teacher believing he is capable of doing so. Amir's teacher notes that lessons involving writing are clear triggers for his outbursts.

On examination in the office, Amir's weight is slightly decreased. He appears irritable and attempts to avoid having his abdomen touched. He winces during the abdominal examination, his abdomen is distended, and some diffuse masses are appreciated.

After a long discussion between the clinician and Amir's parents, the following issues are elucidated:

1. Food selectivity: As with many children on the autism spectrum, Amir has a long history of food selectivity that has worsened as he has gotten older. As formulations for specific commercial foods are changed or eliminated, he has refused replacements and his diet has become more restrictive. It is less likely that a new and medical cause has developed for his increased selectivity, but a high index of suspicion will be maintained if his food selectivity does not improve with a behavioral approach.

   His pediatric primary care clinician believes that he would benefit from outpatient feeding therapy through either a private therapist or an intensive daily feeding program. The family agrees on the need for this intervention and gradually, through the use of food chaining (the gradual introduction of new foods, textures, tastes, and colors based on similarities to preferred foods) and a persistent behavioral approach, the therapist introduces new foods that are closely related to the foods Amir has regularly accepted. The therapist and the parents first work on introducing new brands of strawberry yogurt. They mix the new brand with the old one (after Amir's parents have successfully found the last case within 100 miles). They then proceed to vary the types of pancakes he eats so that, eventually, the family makes his pancakes at home. The family involves Amir in making the pancakes and adding new sources of fiber and food groups into the pancakes. Later, his parents build on the milkshakes he readily drinks and find them to be a good medium for introducing different food groups as well. The parents teach Amir basic information about food groups and nutrition and allow him to make choices and become more involved with shopping and meal preparation. The family sits down weekly to plan and make visual charts for new foods and recipes to introduce.

2. Nutrition: All screening results for anemia, vitamin B_{12}, and zinc deficiencies are negative, and because of the lack of variety in the diet, the primary clinician recommends the use of a multivitamin and additional fiber to support Amir's nutrition. The clinician suggests that the family initiate a program for regular exercise as well. Amir will have regular meetings with a nutritionist, who will provide suggestions for introducing a

variety of whole foods, including fiber-rich options, into his diet. The nutritionist will provide healthy recipes and guidance on food choices to help incorporate these new foods, in collaboration with the feeding therapist.

3. Constipation: Amir has developed progressively worse constipation over the past few years after having established regular toileting behavior in preschool. His poor dietary fiber and fluid intake are thought to be the most likely cause of his constipation, which has progressed to fecal impaction and encopresis. His discomfort with stooling has led to withholding and has compounded the impaction. The primary care clinician introduces a staged approach to treatment. The initial focus is on disimpaction, followed by a long-term maintenance period. The maintenance phase requires the use of laxatives and/or stool softeners; an increase in dietary fiber, fluids, and exercise; and a behavior plan. A daily positive incentive plan for toilet sitting and Valsalva maneuver practice is introduced by Amir's primary care clinician, and other behavioral barriers are addressed by his behavioral therapist.
4. Disruptive behavior: In Amir's case, the behavior is complex. Amir has increased discomfort, chronic constipation, and encopresis. Additionally, a new and challenging task has been introduced in the classroom and his disruptive behavior has been rewarded by allowing him to leave the room, avoid the task, and walk the halls. In addition to addressing the medical causes of his irritability with his primary care clinician, his parents have discussions with a behavioral specialist and his educator that result in their significantly reducing the expectations for his written goals and watching for early signs of stress. The OT makes recommendations for a slanted table and pencil grip that should make writing less taxing. Amir is rewarded for his attempts at writing. His hard work is recognized with breaks, and he is taught to learn to ask for help before he becomes overwhelmed. Over time, Amir becomes less resistant to written work and shows consistent improvement in this area. His behavioral outbursts become less frequent after this multitiered plan is introduced.

Children on the spectrum are at risk for a complexity of GI problems that may be intrinsic to their autism or occur as secondary medical conditions. Many times, the approach to these GI issues requires a clinician to elicit a clear history and approach the most likely cause of the symptoms first, while following the child and monitoring their response to treatment. The chronic issues are likely related to underlying tendencies, but the clinician must remain alert to the existence of red flag signs and symptoms that may reflect the development of a secondary organic etiology.

As is demonstrated in this chapter's case vignette, GI symptoms can be chronic with superimposed secondary issues that require a coordinated multidisciplinary assessment and treatment plan involving the medical team, the educational team, and behavioral specialists. The pediatric primary care clinician should coordinate this care and support the family as they advocate for a comprehensive plan with the school team. This team should ideally include an autism behavioral specialist.

In the case vignette, restrictive eating was related to Amir's underlying sensory issues with eating that were not fully addressed earlier. They became progressively more significant as he further limited the variety of foods he would eat. His constipation became more severe and resulted in fecal withholding, impaction, and incontinence accompanied by pain and distress. This led to diffuse irritability at a time when the school was introducing a new academic demand that was very stressful for Amir. Amir was identified as having effortful and inefficient handwriting skills and was avoidant of this demand when the teacher introduced it as an educational goal. His avoidance behavior was disruptive, and because his teacher allowed him to leave the classroom, she inadvertently reinforced and provided secondary gain for this behavior. Once the medical causes of his irritability were treated and the school recognized that handwriting was a trigger for his behavior, a coordinated positive behavior plan was put into place. The teacher initially lessened the demand for his handwriting, and as he became more able to write and complete these tasks, the educational team was able to further increase the amount of writing he could attend to. If Amir was resistant to a specific demand, the school addressed the source of his resistance and ensured that he returned to the demand with the support needed to be successful. Last, there was an emphasis on teaching Amir to find a way to communicate and express his feelings of being overwhelmed.

Clinical Pearls

- Gastrointestinal disorders often co-occur with sleep disorders, feeding challenges, and/or irritability in children on the autism spectrum.
- Behavioral changes suggestive of possible GI cause are increases in repetitive behaviors, throat clearing, whining, crying, echoing statements about the stomach, agitation, aggression, self-injurious behavior, and task avoidance.
- The prevalence of GI symptoms in children on the spectrum is highly variable.
- Up to 75% of children on the spectrum have GI concerns.
- No GI disease is specific to autism.
- Children on the spectrum tend to have less variety in their diet, so the use of a multivitamin with zinc, vitamin D, and calcium may be warranted after a careful dietary history is elicited.
- The pediatric primary care clinician is the medical home and should coordinate a treatment plan with autism therapists and the educational team.

Parent Resources: Gastrointestinal Issues in Children on the Autism Spectrum

- Autism Speaks. *Parent's Guide to Feeding Behavior in Children with Autism.* 2018. Accessed March 2, 2026. https://www.autismspeaks.org/sites/default/files/2018-08/Exploring%20Feeding%20Behavior.pdf
- Autism Speaks. *Parent's Guide to Managing Constipation in Children with Autism.* 2018. Accessed March 2, 2026. https://www.autismspeaks.org/sites/default/files/2018-08/Constipation%20Guide.pdf
- Ernsperger L, Stegen-Hanson T. *Just Take a Bite: Easy, Effective Answers to Food Aversions and Eating Challenges!* Future Horizons; 2004
- Fraker C, Fishbein M, Coz S, Walbert L. *Food Chaining: The Proven 6-Step Plan to Stop Picky Eating, Solve Feeding Problems, and Expand Your Child's Diet.* Perseus Books Group; 2007
- Reeves PT, Waasdorp Hurtado C. Constipation in children. HealthyChildren.org. July 10, 2024. Accessed March 2, 2026. https://www.healthychildren.org/English/health-issues/conditions/abdominal/Pages/constipation.aspx
- Satter E. *How to Get Your Kid to Eat...but Not Too Much: From Birth to Adolescence.* Bull Publishing Co; 1987
- Williams KE, Foxx RM. *Treating Eating Problems of Children with Autism Spectrum Disorders and Developmental Disabilities.* Pro-Ed: 2007

References

Buie T, Campbell DB, Fuchs GJ III, et al. Evaluation, diagnosis, and treatment of gastrointestinal disorders in individuals with ASDs: a consensus report. *Pediatrics.* 2010;125(suppl 1):S1–S18 PMID: 20048083 doi: 10.1542/peds.2009-1878C

Dhaliwal KK, Orsso CE, Richard C, Haqq AM, Zwaigenbaum L. Risk factors for unhealthy weight gain and obesity among children with autism spectrum disorder. *Int J Mol Sci.* 2019;20(13):3285 PMID: 31277383 doi: 10.3390/ijms20133285

Elder JH. The gluten-free, casein-free diet in autism: an overview with clinical implications. *Nutr Clin Pract.* 2008;23(6):583–588 PMID: 19033217 doi: 10.1177/0884533608326061

Furuta GT, Williams K, Kooros K, et al. Management of constipation in children and adolescents with autism spectrum disorders. *Pediatrics.* 2012;130(suppl 2):S98–S105 PMID: 23118260 doi: 10.1542/peds.2012-0900H

Hyman SL, Levy SE, Myers SM; American Academy of Pediatrics Council on Children With Disabilities and Section on Developmental and Behavioral Pediatrics. Identification, evaluation, and management of children with autism spectrum disorder. *Pediatrics.* 2020;145(1):e20193447 PMID: 31843864 doi: 10.1542/peds.2019-3447

Hyman SL, Stewart PA, Foley J, et al. The gluten-free/casein-free diet: a double-blind challenge trial in children with autism. *J Autism Dev Disord.* 2016;46(1):205–220 PMID: 26343026 doi: 10.1007/s10803-015-2564-9

Keller A, Rimestad ML, Friis Rohde J, et al. The effect of a combined gluten- and casein-free diet on children and adolescents with autism spectrum disorders: a systematic review and meta-analysis. *Nutrients.* 2021;13(2):470 PMID: 33573238 doi: 10.3390/nu13020470

Leader G, Abberton C, Cunningham S, et al. Gastrointestinal symptoms in autism spectrum disorder: a systematic review. *Nutrients.* 2022;14(7):1471 PMID: 35406084 doi: 10.3390/nu14071471

Lyall K, Van de Water J, Ashwood P, Hertz-Picciotto I. Asthma and allergies in children with autism spectrum disorders: results from the CHARGE study. *Autism Res.* 2015;8(5):567–574 PMID: 25722050 doi: 10.1002/aur.1471

Smile S, Raffaele C, Perlin R. Re-imagining the physicians' role in the assessment of feeding challenges in children with autism spectrum disorder. *Paediatr Child Health.* 2020;26(2):e73–e77 PMID: 34484495 doi: 10.1093/pch/pxaa008

Xu G, Snetselaar LG, Jing J, Liu B, Strathearn L, Bao W. Association of food allergy and other allergic conditions with autism spectrum disorder in children. *JAMA Netw Open.* 2018;1(2):e180279 PMID: 30646068 doi: 10.1001/jamanetworkopen.2018.0279

CHAPTER

12

Insomnia: Identification and Interventions

CASE VIGNETTE

Addi is a 4-year-old-child on the autism spectrum. She is a delightful child who is active, is often emotionally dysregulated, and can be difficult to soothe. Addi attends full-time preschool and naps from 3:00 to 5:00 pm. When she comes home at 5:00 pm, her family of 5 is engaged in preparing dinner, completing homework, tidying the house, bathing, and then getting ready for bed. The bedtime routine is chaotic, as Addi's parents have to balance her needs with those of her 2 siblings. Addi's parents focus on getting her younger siblings to bed first, as Addi will not sit for a bedtime story. When Addi's parents try to put her to bed, she becomes more active while happily singing her favorite song. She repeatedly runs from her bedroom to watch her favorite video, and her parents inevitably tire and allow her to fall asleep next to them on the couch after 10:00 pm. Later they move her to her own bed while she is asleep. Addi is difficult to wake at 6:45 am, and the morning routine is stressful.

Addi is described as a restless sleeper who flips around in her bed. She does not snore and sleeps through the night on most nights. She does, however, awaken 2 to 3 nights per week and requires her parents to come into her room repeatedly to help her settle before she returns to sleep. Sometimes Addi's parents allow her to sleep with them. On the weekends, Addi sleeps several hours later than during the week, and she tends to fall asleep in the car when the family goes on outings. Addi is able to eat independently while joining the family at mealtime. She has a very limited dietary repertoire and prefers dairy products and carbohydrates. She eats no meat and few vegetables. The family seeks advice from their pediatric primary care clinician about how to encourage more healthy sleep for Addi and the family.

The pediatric clinician is often called on to answer parent concerns about their children's sleep. The significance of the effects of sleep disorders on family functioning and well-being and the availability of the child for learning and prosocial behavior are well-documented. In the context of autism, insomnia is not only more frequent, occurring in 53% to 78% of those on the spectrum compared to 26% to 32% of typically developing children, but has effects that can lead both to a higher level of difficulty around the expression of core features of autism and to daytime externalizing and disruptive behaviors. Insomnia not only significantly affects children and their families but tends to persist into adulthood in 50% of individuals.

Insomnia is defined by Malow and colleagues as any "repeated difficulty with sleep initiation, duration, consolidation, or quality that occurs despite age-appropriate time and opportunity for sleep." Despite the prevalence of sleep disruptions and their effect on the child and the family, sleep issues in children on the spectrum are underreported by parents and underidentified by clinicians. A systematic approach to evaluating sleep is important, and this chapter offers an approach and algorithm for assessing and treating insomnia in the autistic child.

Screening for Sleep Issues

It is recommended that all children on the autism spectrum be screened routinely for insomnia. Screening for sleep problems in the autistic child is no different from that in the typically developing child except for the increased likelihood of related co-occurring medical conditions in children on the spectrum. There are 2 sleep screeners regularly used to better define sleep patterns. These provide a helpful structure to screening and identify contributors to insomnia that will serve to guide the treatment plan. The BEARS sleep screening tool (**Box 12.1**) is a simple acronym that is used to help prompt the clinician to remember the relevant historical information to collect: **B**edtime problems, **E**xcessive daytime sleepiness, **A**wakenings during the night, **R**egularity of sleep schedule, and **S**leep-disordered breathing. The screener can be administered to a parent or caregiver, or the clinician can use these prompts when eliciting a history.

The Children's Sleep Habits Questionnaire (CSHQ) is a more extensive parent-report questionnaire that is available as a shortened 22-item form, the Short-Form CSHQ (SF-CSHQ) (**Figure 12.1**). The more complete tool was developed with a population of typically developing children, making some items potentially irrelevant to a child on the spectrum. The shortened form presented here has more relevance to a population with developmental differences such as autism.

BOX 12.1 The BEARS Sleep Screening Tool

Bedtime problems: Does child struggle going to sleep?

Excessive daytime sleepiness: Is child sleepy during the day? Does the child fall asleep during the day?

Awakenings during the night: Does child wake up during the night?

Regularity of sleep: Does child have predictable bedtime and wake-up times?

Sleep-disordered breathing: Does child snore or have difficulty breathing during night?

Adapted with permission from Owens JA, Dalzell V. Use of the "BEARS" sleep screening tool in a pediatric residents' continuity clinic: a pilot study. *Sleep Medicine.* 2005;6(1):63–69.

The SF-CSHQ collects more detailed information about sleep patterns, sleep associations, routines, sleep behaviors, and daytime sleepiness, as well as the presence of specific signs indicative of primary sleep disorders (obstructive sleep apnea, night terrors, nightmares, and restless legs syndrome [RLS]).

Screening for Medical Etiologies

As discussed in earlier chapters, insomnia can be a primary disorder or a manifestation of underlying medical etiologies. Most insomnias in children are behavioral in etiology. As a result, a clinician's involvement in teaching parents to set clear, predictable bedtime routines is critical and will be addressed in the Nonpharmacological Treatments section later in this chapter. An excellent literature review and practice pathway specific to insomnia in children and adolescents on the autism spectrum was developed by Malow and colleagues as part of the Sleep Committee of the Autism Treatment Network (ATN). This group created a parent insomnia toolkit that is available on the Autism Speaks website (www.autismspeaks.org/sites/default/files/2018-08/Sleep%20Tool%20Kit.pdf). The practice pathway recommends that clinicians screen all children on the spectrum for insomnia, consider medical etiologies, and recommend behavioral interventions before pharmacological agents are considered.

When evaluating sleep disturbances in children on the spectrum, a comprehensive history for medical issues that could cause or exacerbate sleep disturbances should be performed. The review should include symptoms suggestive of gastroesophageal reflux disease (GERD), constipation, abdominal or other pain sources, or seizures;

The following statements are about your child's sleep habits and possible difficulties with sleep. Think about the past week in your life when you answer the questions. If last week was unusual for a specific reason, choose the most recent typical week. Unless noted, check Always if something occurs every night, Usually if it occurs 5 or 6 times a week, Sometimes if it occurs 2 to 4 times a week, Rarely if it occurs once a week, and Never if it occurs less than once a week.

BEDTIME

Write in your child's usual bedtime: Weeknights ______ : ______ am/pm
Weekends ______ : ______ am/pm

	7 Always	5–6 Usually	2–4 Sometimes	1 Rarely	0 Never
1. Child goes to bed at the same time at night.	( )	( )	( )	( )	( )
2. Child falls asleep within 20 minutes after going to bed.	( )	( )	( )	( )	( )
3. Child falls asleep alone in own bed.	( )	( )	( )	( )	( )
4. Child falls asleep in parent's or sibling's bed.	( )	( )	( )	( )	( )
5. Child falls asleep with rocking or rhythmic movements.	( )	( )	( )	( )	( )
6. Child needs special object to fall asleep (doll, special blanket, stuffed animal, etc).	( )	( )	( )	( )	( )
7. Child needs parent in the room to fall asleep.	( )	( )	( )	( )	( )
8. Child resists going to bed at bedtime.	( )	( )	( )	( )	( )
9. Child is afraid of sleeping in the dark.	( )	( )	( )	( )	( )

SLEEP BEHAVIOR

Write in your child's usual amount of sleep each day
(combining nighttime sleep and naps): ______ hours and ______ minutes

	7 Always	5–6 Usually	2–4 Sometimes	1 Rarely	0 Never
10. Child sleeps about the same amount each day.	( )	( )	( )	( )	( )
11. Child is restless and moves a lot during sleep.	( )	( )	( )	( )	( )
12. Child moves to someone else's bed during the night (parent, sibling, etc).	( )	( )	( )	( )	( )
13. Child grinds teeth during sleep (your dentist may have told you this).	( )	( )	( )	( )	( )
14. Child snores loudly.	( )	( )	( )	( )	( )
15. Child awakens during the night and is sweating, screaming, and inconsolable.	( )	( )	( )	( )	( )
16. Child naps during the day.	( )	( )	( )	( )	( )

Write in the number of minutes the nap usually lasts: ______ minutes

WAKING DURING THE NIGHT

	7 Always	5–6 Usually	2–4 Sometimes	1 Rarely	0 Never
17. Child wakes up once during the night.	( )	( )	( )	( )	( )
18. Child wakes up more than once during the night.	( )	( )	( )	( )	( )

MORNING WAKE UP

Write in the time child usually wakes up in the morning: Weekdays ______ : ______ am/pm
Weekends ______ : ______ am/pm

	7 Always	5–6 Usually	2–4 Sometimes	1 Rarely	0 Never
19. Child wakes up by him/herself.	( )	( )	( )	( )	( )
20. Child wakes up very early in the morning (or, earlier than necessary or desired).	( )	( )	( )	( )	( )
21. Child seems tired during the daytime.	( )	( )	( )	( )	( )
22. Child falls asleep while involved in activities.	( )	( )	( )	( )	( )

A score above 30 indicates a pediatric sleep disorder.

Figure 12.1. Short-Form Children's Sleep Habits Questionnaire

Adapted with permission from Owens JA, Spirito A, McGuinn M. The Children's Sleep Habits Questionnaire (CSHQ): psychometric properties of a survey instrument for school-aged children. *Sleep.* 2000;23(8):1043–1051.

risk factors for low iron stores; and evidence of obstructive sleep apnea or other breathing problems, asthma, and/or pruritus, in addition to sleep associations. The practice pathway provides a useful screening tool to assist in this detailed review of possible causative factors of insomnia. Refer to **Figure 12.2** for a checklist of medical contributors to insomnia. If the insomnia persists after addressing all possible medical factors, the treatment should focus on behavioral interventions.

Neurobiological Causes

Some individuals on the autism spectrum have abnormal sleep architecture compared to typically developing peers. Different types of atypical sleep patterns have been reported, including prolonged sleep latency, reduced total sleep time, and reduced rapid eye movement (REM) and non-REM sleep. These findings suggest a neurobiological etiology for the sleep disorder, and the neurotransmitters γ-aminobutyric acid (GABA), serotonin, and melatonin have been implicated. Unfortunately, aside from the use of melatonin (discussed in the Pharmacological Treatments section later in this chapter), these potential neurochemical links to atypical sleep in the setting of autism have not yet resulted in effective pharmacological treatments.

GABA is an inhibitory neurotransmitter that is involved in sleep onset as well as behavioral inhibition. The theory is that decreased GABA levels result in both

Check the appropriate response or write in the parent's response as indicated.		
Gastrointestinal	**Yes**	**No**
1. Does your child have a history of reflux? • *If yes, has it resolved?* • *If yes, when did it resolve?*	☐ ☐	☐ ☐
2. Are there any ongoing symptoms? • *If yes, list all:*	☐	☐
3. Does your child have constipation? • *If yes, is it controlled?* • *What medication(s) is(are) used for control?*	☐ ☐	☐ ☐
4. Does your child have abdominal pain? 5. Does it occur at night? • *If yes, how often does it occur?*	☐ ☐	☐ ☐
Seizures and other nighttime events	**Yes**	**No**
1. Does your child have seizures? • *If yes, does your child have seizures that happen multiple times a night?*	☐ ☐	☐ ☐
2. Does your child have unusual events (behaviors or movements) during the night? • *If yes, is the event similar every time (suggests seizure)?*	☐ ☐	☐ ☐
Sleep-disordered breathing	**Yes**	**No**
1. Does your child snore/breathe loudly?	☐	☐
2. Does your child gasp for breath or stop breathing? (If no, the child may still have sleep-disordered breathing.)	☐	☐
3. Does your child have allergies/nasal congestion?	☐	☐
Asthma/sinusitis	**Yes**	**No**
1. Does your child cough at night?	☐	☐
Pain/itching/discomfort	**Yes**	**No**
1. Does your child see a dentist regularly?	☐	☐
2. Could your child have any tooth pain?	☐	☐
3. Does your child have eczema? • *If your child has eczema, is it currently well controlled?* • *What medication is used for controlling the eczema?* • *When is the medication used (ie, daily, as needed)?* • *Do you think that the eczema causes your child to be itchy or have pain?*	☐ ☐ ☐	☐ ☐ ☐
4. Could your child be hungry at night?	☐	☐
5. Is your child overly sensitive to light, sounds, or textures of clothing?	☐	☐
6. Can you think of anything that may be causing your child pain? • *If yes, explain:*	☐	☐
Nutrition	**Yes**	**No**
1. Does your child eat at least 1–2 ounces of meat per day?	☐	☐
2. If not, does your child take a multivitamin with iron? • *If yes, how often?*	☐	☐
3. Does your child have restless sleep?	☐	☐
4. Does your child have leg pains/"growing pains"?	☐	☐

Physical examination	Yes	No
1. Does the child have large tonsils?	☐	☐
2. Is the child hypotonic?	☐	☐
3. Does the child have nasal congestion or signs of allergic rhinitis?	☐	☐
4. Does the child have dental issues?	☐	☐
5. Does the child have wheezing?	☐	☐
6. Does the child have significant eczema?	☐	☐

Figure 12.2. Questionnaire to Screen for Underlying Medical Causes of Insomnia

Adapted from Malow BA, Byars K, Johnson K, et al; Sleep Committee of the Autism Treatment Network. A practice pathway for the identification, evaluation, and management of insomnia in children and adolescents with autism spectrum disorders. *Pediatrics.* 2012;130(suppl 2):S106–S124.

hyperarousal and insomnia. Serotonin has also been implicated, as some individuals on the spectrum have been noted to have elevated serotonin levels. This elevation may result in both excessive wakefulness and REM inhibition. Lower levels of melatonin, on the other hand, have been repeatedly demonstrated in those on the spectrum as well as in those with attention-deficit/hyperactivity disorder (ADHD). Melatonin is typically secreted by the pineal gland in response to darkness and aids the transition into sleep. This finding supports the use of melatonin to support sleep latency, and more detail is provided in the Pharmacological Treatments section later in this chapter.

Nonpharmacological Treatments

Behavioral therapy and parent education are always the first and most effective interventions for sleep disruptions for all children. Most children with insomnia respond to behavioral interventions alone, and there are many effective ways a pediatric primary care clinician can offer these strategies. The ATN insomnia toolkit (www.autismspeaks.org/tool-kit/strategies-improve-sleep-children-autism) is an excellent parent teaching aid for behavioral intervention and provides tools such as visual schedules (**Figure 12.3**) and a bedtime pass. Clinicians can share this toolkit with parents to support the family's efforts to achieve healthy sleep. Note that this resource requires a free registration to access the tools.

Parent education for insomnia and bedtime refusal starts with consistent bedtime routines. These strategies are detailed in the following list. A shorter list to share with parents or to use in the medical record (**Box 12.2**) follows, as well as a list of parent resources at the end of this chapter.

- **Predictable bedtime routines:** Teaching parents about the importance of a predictable bedtime and routine supports the healthy establishment of a child's expectations for bedtime and the development of a circadian rhythm. It is this internal circadian rhythm that establishes patterns of sleep and arousal. Further,

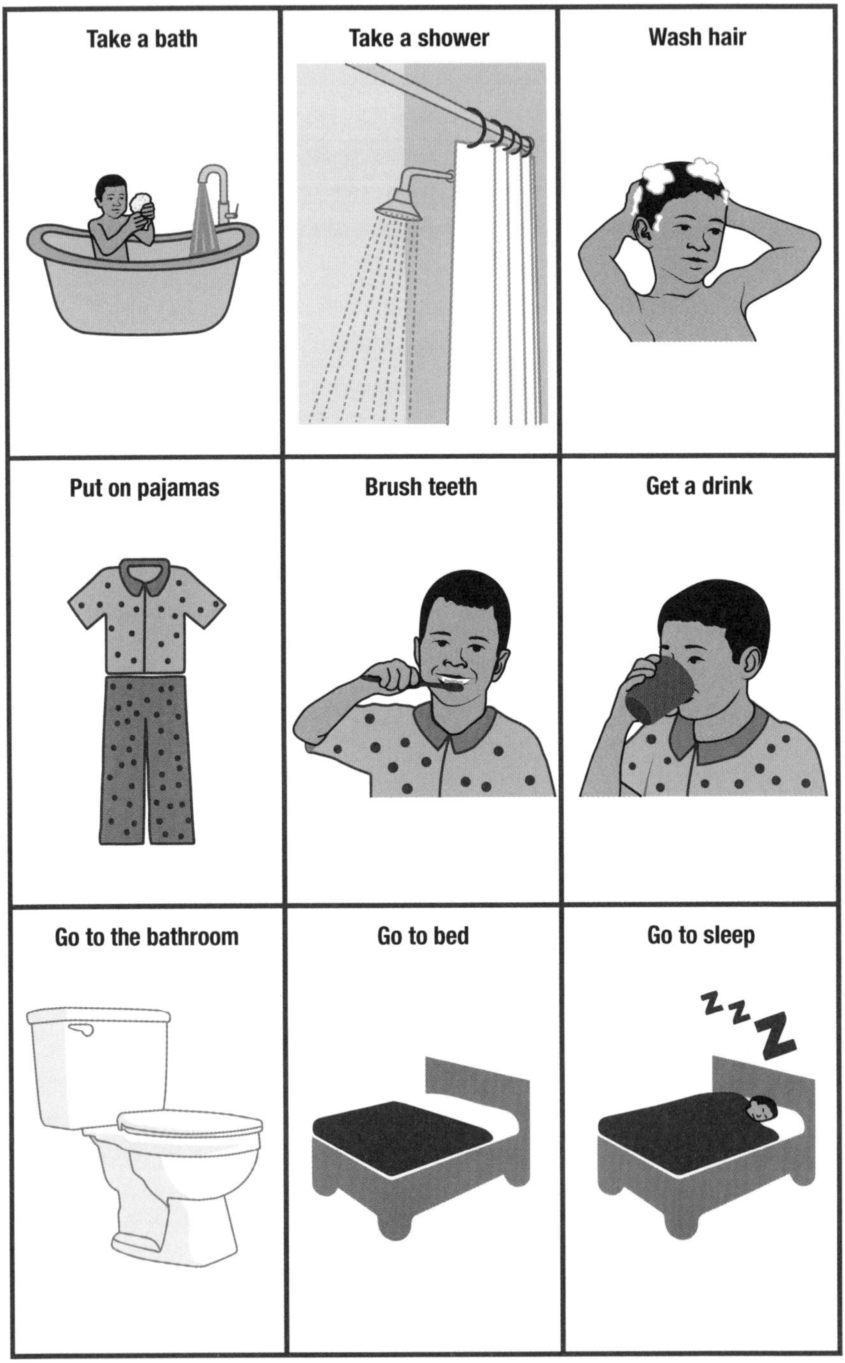
Take a bath
Take a shower
Wash hair
Put on pajamas
Brush teeth
Get a drink
Go to the bathroom
Go to bed
Go to sleep
Z
Z
Z

Figure 12.3. Visual Schedule for Sleep
Adapted from Autism Speaks. *Sleep Strategies for Children with Autism.* 2018. Accessed March 3, 2026. https://www.autismspeaks.org/sites/default/files/2018-08/Sleep%20Tool%20Kit.pdf.

BOX 12.2 Interventions for Sleep Interruptions

Behavioral Interventions for the Parent to Implement

- Establish a predictable, calming bedtime routine.
- Set a wake-up time; allow for resetting of circadian rhythm.
- Teach strategies for self-soothing: breathing, singing a song, and hugging a favorite comfort item (eg, a stuffed toy).
- Maintain a comfortable environment for sleep: keep the temperature between 68 and 72 °F; block out excessive light; remove stimulating toys, activities, and people; and consider use of white noise or a fan.
- Use tools (eg, social stories, visual aids) to support a consistent sleep routine.
- Consider using a 2-way monitor to view the child and provide reassurance without entering the room.
- Adjust sleep associations (eg, gradual extinction of feedings, parent in room).
- Use a bedtime fading strategy: set the bedtime for when the child is falling asleep and gradually move it earlier.
- Eliminate caffeine, the use of screens/devices, and any TV in the bedroom.
- Introduce a behavioral incentive plan to encourage cooperation.
- Consider the use of a bedtime pass.

Medical Interventions for the Clinician to Implement

- Assess for medical contributors (eg, caffeine, alcohol, medications).
- Consider a mental health referral for coexisting conditions (eg, anxiety, depression, obsessive-compulsive disorder).
- Refer for a sleep study/to an otolaryngologist for evidence of obstructive sleep apnea, restless legs syndrome, or persistent symptoms.
- Consider use of melatonin for children not responding to behavioral intervention alone.

consistency in place and routine is essential for the establishment of autonomous sleep transition. This involves consistently putting the child to bed in the same place, with the same associated routines, and leaving the room before the child is asleep. Initiating these routines during infancy will support the early establishment of healthy sleep behavior. The child should not be given a bottle or food to fall asleep and should be able to transition to sleep alone to establish autonomous habits that support falling asleep easily and sleeping through the night.

- **Soothing activities:** Many children on the autism spectrum have sensory needs and self-regulation difficulties that hinder a transition to sleep. Soothing routines may include rocking, singing, reciting nursery rhymes, reading a book, listening to music, using a ceiling fan or white noise machine, doing deep breathing, practicing guided visualization, hugging a comfort item, or wearing tight clothing or bedclothes to aid calming and the transition to sleep.

(Suggestions involving soft objects and materials should be made only to families that have children older than 12 months to avoid suffocation risk.) Parents can introduce and model these activities so the child can learn to independently self-soothe while falling asleep. Consultation with an occupational therapist may be helpful if the parents seek further guidance and specific strategies. Parents should observe which activities increase the child's arousal and learn to avoid these as a part of bedtime, including physical activity, screen exposure, or foods or medications containing stimulants (eg, caffeine). Further, parents should be advised to dress the child lightly and keep the room temperature between 68 and 72 °F.

- **Social stories and visual aids:** Children with communication challenges may respond more robustly when a visual representation of the expectations and routines is used, and the child's therapist or educator might assist with creating these tools. Clinicians can refer parents to the Autism Speaks toolkit *Sleep Strategies for Children with Autism* (www.autismspeaks.org/sites/default/files/2018-08/Sleep%20Tool%20Kit.pdf) for examples. Refer to **Figure 12.3** for an example of a visual aid to support sleep routines.
- **Positive behavior intervention:** Positive reinforcement with intrinsically motivating rewards (an extra snuggle or an extra book) can be used to encourage the child to follow the bedtime routine without resistance. Praise and acknowledgment of the child's successes foster confidence and encourage further success. A bedtime pass can be effective with an older child who has adequate communication skills to understand instruction. The bedtime pass is a physical document that is given to the child at bedtime. The child is told they can use the pass only once, to leave their room or call for help, while going to sleep. Alternatively, the child can choose to hold on to the pass while falling asleep independently. If successful, the child can exchange the pass for a highly motivating reward the next morning (a special privilege or breakfast treat). It should be clarified that if the child is ill or in distress, they can always call for help.
- **Gradual extinction:** Gradual extinction is a technique used to wean a child from dependency on the parent's presence or actions to fall asleep. When children depend on the parent for sleep transition, they may wake the parent if they come to arousal between sleep cycles. Examples include the parent lying down with the child, giving the child a bottle to fall asleep, and responding to delaying tactics (eg, trips to the bathroom). The clinician will need to review with parents how to wean a child from such a dependency for the child to be able to initiate and maintain sleep independently. Sudden removal of these behaviors can elicit protests and additional sleep interruptions. Some parents may prefer to stop the associated behavior altogether and address any resulting protests, but most prefer a gradual program. If a parent resorts to lying down with the child, clinicians can instruct them to sit at the child's side and gradually, over days,

move farther away from the child until they are sitting outside the child's door. Similarly with bedtime or trained nighttime feeding, the transition may be easier if the milk is diluted or the amount of liquid or snack offered is gradually decreased and the child therefore experiences less hunger at this time. Parents should be instructed that healthy toddlers and older children do not need food at bedtime or during the night and are able to adjust their caloric intake to the daytime. Once extinction of association is achieved and the child has developed the skills to fall asleep independently, they will be more successful at putting themselves back to sleep during the night. It is important to be certain there is no secondary gain to night waking, such as screen watching, playing, or eating.

- **Bedtime fading:** Children who have protracted bedtime routines and fall asleep late in the night should have the new bedtime routine introduced at the time when they are already falling asleep. The parent is more likely to be successful if they make these behavioral changes at this later time. They can then gradually move the bedtime routine to a more age-appropriate time.

When behavioral interventions are ineffective or when there are signs of underlying issues, it is essential to conduct a thorough assessment for any co-occurring behavioral health concerns. If necessary, a referral to a psychiatrist or therapist may be appropriate to address these issues.

For children who exhibit snoring, who have symptoms suggestive of obstructive sleep apnea, or who are not responding to initial treatment, a referral to an otolaryngologist or a sleep specialist may be warranted. A sleep study can help identify the specific nature of the child's disrupted sleep and assess for conditions such as RLS or periodic limb movement disorder (PLMD). These data will help inform necessary next steps in intervention.

Pharmacological Treatments

There are no US Food and Drug Administration (FDA)–approved medications for the management of insomnia in children on or not on the autism spectrum. There is adequate documentation that melatonin is effective and safe for short-term use in children older than 3 years. Melatonin is considered a nutritional supplement and, as a result, is not regulated by the FDA. Parents should be encouraged to use the same brand consistently, cautioned about the risk for ingestion, and reminded to store all medication and supplements out of the child's reach. Additionally, melatonin should be used only for the child with sleep-onset insomnia and after all possible medical causes have been addressed. Clinicians can inform parents that there is a lack of research on the long-term use of melatonin and should encourage short-term use. The risk of increasing seizure threshold as well as the pragmatics of dosing should be reviewed. Instructions should include starting at a low dose of 0.5 mg and slowly titrating it if needed, up to 5 or 6 mg, given 30 to 45 minutes before desired sleep onset as a onetime dose. There are many formulations of melatonin, and some families will be unaware of the difference between measurement in volume and the actual amount of medication (milliliter/mL versus milligram/mg). It is recommended that a parent bring the medication or a photo of the bottle to review with the clinician at the follow-up visit.

There is an association between low iron stores and RLS, and treatment can bring positive results in sleep interruption. In the child with persistent nighttime waking, the clinician should check a serum ferritin level and, if the level is less than 50 ng/mL, treat it with supplemental iron and possible diet changes, with follow-up in 3 months. The child's ferritin level should be checked as needed until it is above 50 ng/mL and their insomnia symptoms resolve. If there is further concern for RLS and/or PLMD, the child should be referred to a sleep specialist for evaluation.

Other autistic children with associated co-occurring behavioral health conditions tend to have concurrent improvement in sleep when the behavioral health condition is treated with either pharmacological or behavioral interventions. For example, an autistic child with coexisting aggression and irritability may be prescribed an atypical neuroleptic (risperidone or aripiprazole), which may also treat the sleep disorder. An autistic child with depression, anxiety, or ADHD may have better sleep when the underlying behavioral health condition is treated. Both trazodone and mirtazapine can ease the symptoms of depression and the insomnia and may be chosen when depression is present. Similarly, as has been observed with neurotypical children, when ADHD and anxiety symptoms are treated with medication in children on the spectrum, bedtime and settling issues are likely to improve as well.

After evaluation, if no clear etiology of insomnia has been identified and/or interventions are unsuccessful, the child should be referred to a sleep specialist. A sleep study may be warranted to evaluate for obstructive sleep apnea or other sleep disorders. If the child cannot tolerate a sleep study and they are snoring, a referral to an otolaryngologist to evaluate tonsils and adenoids may be warranted.

CASE VIGNETTE: CONCLUSION

The case of Addi presents many of the sleep-associated difficulties the pediatric primary care clinician is likely to encounter in children on the autism spectrum: erratic sleep schedule, sleep associations that promote a dependence on the presence of others to fall asleep, difficulty self-soothing to settle at bedtime, and concern for possible RLS. There are no concerns raised for other possible medical contributors such as obstructive sleep apnea, constipation, GERD, or sources of pain or discomfort.

On consultation with the pediatric primary clinician, Addi's parents develop a sleep treatment plan as follows:

- A consistent bedtime routine using fading and extinction: Addi's parents first initiate her bedtime routine at 10:00 pm, when she has already been falling asleep. Since the other children are already asleep at this time, one of the adults sits with Addi and introduces some sensory routines that are soothing to her: rocking in a chair, singing a familiar song together, cuddling with a favorite object, and tucking her bedclothes in tightly. They then leave the room while Addi is sleepy but still awake and may need to return to help her settle. They no longer stay in the room until she falls asleep or allow her to co-sleep.Once Addi's routine is established, her parents gradually fade her bedtime back to a more reasonable hour in 15-minute increments. Addi's parents insist on her staying in her bedroom without a screen. Her parents find that the first month of sleep training is more effective when they give her 1 mg of melatonin 1 hour before bedtime, but once her sleep habits have improved, they no longer find it necessary to continue the melatonin.
- An assessment for medical contributors: Given the concern for RLS, a serum ferritin test is ordered and Addi's level is found to be low. Oral iron therapy is initiated while Addi's parents receive nutritional guidance to increase her consumption of iron-containing foods and decrease her consumption of dairy products to an average amount.
- Follow-up: Addi returns in 3 months and her parents report dramatic improvement. Addi will now fall asleep alone after a consistent bedtime routine. She only occasionally requires her parents to reenter her bedroom to help her settle. Addi is easier to rouse in the mornings now that her bedtime has been moved slowly back to 8:30 pm and that she gets 10 hours of sleep consistently. Addi's parents request that her afternoon nap at school be started no later than 1:00 pm, and they wake her on weekends at the same time she wakes during the week. Addi's parents and her primary care clinician decide not to check another ferritin level unless her insomnia relapses, and they decide to stop the iron supplements at this time.

Sleep disorders are common and multifactorial in children on the spectrum. All children on the spectrum should undergo regular screening for sleep disorders and will require ongoing monitoring of their progress. Assessing a child for insomnia requires a systematic approach to look for possible medical and behavioral health contributors or etiology. There are screening tools available to assist the pediatric primary care clinician in this assessment. Sleep disorders can have significant and lasting effects on a child's ability to learn and be both socially and academically successful. Sleep disturbances affect families in addition to the child. Most sleep disorders will be behavioral in etiology and will respond to parent education and behavioral intervention initiated by primary care clinicians. The underlying medical contributors must be addressed concurrently, and children who do not respond to primary care management or with signs or symptoms indicative of primary sleep disorders should be referred for specialty assessment and care.

Clinical Pearls

- Insomnias are very common in children on the autism spectrum.
- These insomnias include difficulties with sleep onset, sleep duration, sleep quality, and sleep consolidation.
- Children on the spectrum are more likely to have medical conditions that may be associated with their insomnia.
- Most insomnias respond to behavioral intervention, which can be successfully introduced by the primary care clinician.

Parent Resources: Insomnia and Autism

- Autism Speaks. *How to Use Sleep Strategies to Help Your Child with Autism.* Accessed March 3, 2026. https://www.autismspeaks.org/sites/default/files/SC_ATN%20Sleep%20Topic%20Flyer_083120_v5.pdf
- Autism Speaks. *Sleep Strategies for Children with Autism.* 2018. Accessed March 3, 2026. https://www.autismspeaks.org/sites/default/files/2018-08/Sleep%20Tool%20Kit.pdf

References

Buckley AW, Hirtz D, Oskoui M, et al. Practice guideline: treatment for insomnia and disrupted sleep behavior in children and adolescents with autism spectrum disorder: report of the Guideline Development, Dissemination, and Implementation Subcommittee of the American Academy of Neurology. *Neurology.* 2020;94(9):392–404 PMID: 32051244 doi: 10.1212/WNL.0000000000009033

Galli J, Loi E, Visconti LM, et al; ASD Collaborative Group. Sleep disturbances in children affected by autism spectrum disorder. *Front Psychiatry.* 2022;13:736696 PMID: 35250655 doi: 10.3389/fpsyt.2022.736696

Johnson KP, Zarrinnegar P. Autism spectrum disorder and sleep. *Child Adolesc Psychiatr Clin N Am.* 2021;30(1):195–208 PMID: 33223062 doi: 10.1016/j.chc.2020.08.012

Malow BA, Byars K, Johnson K, et al; Sleep Committee of the Autism Treatment Network. A practice pathway for the identification, evaluation, and management of insomnia in children and adolescents with autism spectrum disorders. *Pediatrics.* 2012;130(suppl 2):S106–S124 PMID: 23118242 doi: 10.1542/peds.2012-0900I

Mindell JA, Kuhn B, Lewin DS, Meltzer LJ, Sadeh A; American Academy of Sleep Medicine. Behavioral treatment of bedtime problems and night wakings in infants and young children. *Sleep.* 2006;29(10):1263–1276 PMID: 17068979

CHAPTER 13

Review of Pharmacotherapy and Complementary Interventions

CASE VIGNETTE

Eva is a fun-loving, active 8-year-old child on the autism spectrum. Since diagnosis in preschool, Eva has attended self-contained autism education programs. Over the years, her communication skills have improved and, with one-on-one instruction, she has made developmental strides. In first grade, she was happy to learn letters and begin phonics in the general education class while spending the remainder of her day in an autism self-contained classroom. Her individualized education program (IEP) focuses on issues related to her restricted and repetitive behaviors (RRBs) and irritability. She can easily be triggered by a request to transition or an academic task that is not a preferred activity. Her parents additionally note that with many daily tasks and demands, Eva becomes dysregulated and has a tantrum. Her irritability and emotional outbursts have continued to worsen in second grade. Now Eva is often frustrated. She may push or hit a peer who reaches for something she seeks, and she struggles with turn taking. In the general education classroom, she may yell out when someone does something she does not like, and her outbursts in school and at home have become more frequent. Her parents struggle with the evening routine, including getting her to settle for sleep. They have removed many classroom demands and allow her to play alone instead. They find she may now spontaneously have a tantrum and has begun to throw or hit others, including her sibling. In the school setting, the teacher has had to remove the other children when she was unable to calm Eva. The frequency and intensity of these outbursts are increasing, and Eva's teacher and school staff have expressed their concern to Eva's parents.

In the course of caring for a child on the spectrum, the primary care clinician will often be asked by their patient's caregivers to consider whether there is an indication for psychopharmacological intervention. Although there are no medications shown to effectively treat the core features of autism if they begin to interfere with functioning, medication use can be helpful when addressing many of the co-occurring behavioral health concerns. As discussed in previous chapters, autism is an extremely heterogeneous entity and there is no single recommendation that is applicable to all children and adolescents. Not only should each child, family, school placement, and level of intervention be considered, but a thorough understanding of the research literature on the use of pharmacological agents for each indication is helpful and addressed in this chapter. As discussed in Chapter 10, Diagnosing and Managing Co-Occurring Conditions, individuals on the spectrum frequently present with additional medical and behavioral health conditions. Medical conditions such as insomnia, gastrointestinal (GI) distress, allergies, and dental pain, as well as medication adverse effects, can present with behavioral manifestations in an individual who may not be able to communicate what they are experiencing. The necessity of a careful behavior analysis to identify underlying triggers to new behavioral concerns and to determine which supports and treatment goals are indicated has also been explored in previous chapters. A new teacher, a new classroom placement, a seating placement next to a child who might trigger a reaction, a specific experience or sensory exposure that might trigger anxiety, a challenging demand, stress over a school exam, or conflict at home can all contribute to irritability, hyperactivity, or emotional dysregulation. Prioritizing behavioral interventions and accommodations and evaluating their efficacy should be the first tier of support, and medication treatment should be adjunctive and secondary. Further, children on the spectrum are more susceptible to adverse effects, including *activation* (induced agitation), from psychotropic medications, making it important to prescribe medications carefully.

The pediatric primary care clinician is positioned to be the professional best able to witness a child's developmental progression, assess evolving concerns and their contributors, and intervene early. In consultation with specialists, the primary care clinician should determine when medication introduction may be necessary while assessing the effects of first-line therapies and weighing the risks and benefits for each child's profile. It is not expected that all pediatric clinicians develop expertise in every aspect of psychopharmaceutical intervention. Rather, it is expected that the pediatric primary care clinician have familiarity with use of these medications and when to refer to specialists who can assume care of the child for whom medication management is indicated.

Becoming familiar with both the indications for initiating medication and the available pharmacological agents is an essential first step. It has become increasingly important for the pediatric primary care clinician to develop this expertise, as access to developmental-behavioral pediatricians and/or psychiatrists has become progressively more challenging for families. Many pediatric primary care clinicians will initiate a first-line medication trial and will refer patients to developmental-behavioral pediatricians or psychiatrists if their initial introduction of medication is ineffective and/or poorly tolerated. This threshold for referral will vary with experience, but ideally the pediatric primary care clinician will have enough expertise to be able to initiate a medication trial and develop increasing levels of competence as they learn to care for children on the spectrum. Sharing the care of these children with experienced specialists can support the clinician's educational process and practice. Pediatric clinicians in most states have access to teleconsultation services to obtain guidance from psychiatrists. The state-sponsored Pediatric Mental Health Care Access Program recipients that provide pediatric clinicians with telephone consultations and often with additional educational resources are listed on the Maternal and Child Health Bureau website (https://mchb.hrsa.gov/programs-impact/programs/pmhca-awardee-teleconsultation-phone-lines). The American Academy of Child and Adolescent Psychiatry (AACAP) has many live and online courses on autism care management and the use of psychopharmacological agents (www.aacap.org/AACAP/CME_and_Meetings/CME/Online_CME.aspx). The American Academy of Pediatrics (AAP) has ample resources to support the pediatric primary care clinician learning about autism care management and psychopharmacology, including *Pediatric Psychopharmacology for Primary Care,* 4th Edition. Additionally, the AACAP has available a series of Parents' Medication Guides developed in collaboration with the American Psychiatric Association that offer up-to-date information about medication prescribing related to attention-deficit/hyperactivity disorder (ADHD), anxiety, bipolar disorders, depression, autism, and insomnia (www.aacap.org/AACAP/Families_Youth/Parents_Medication_Guides/AACAP/Families_and_Youth/Family_Resources/Parents_Medication_Guides.aspx).

The Research

There are solid research data based on prospective randomized controlled studies and clinical experience that help guide the process of identifying indications and choosing psychopharmacological agents. Each decision requires an analysis of possible risks and benefits. Medications carry different risks for adverse effects, and many children on the autism spectrum seem to be particularly vulnerable to these effects. For this reason, it is important that medication use be considered only after medical contributors have been addressed and a thorough assessment of behavioral triggers has been analyzed. For the autistic child, it is particularly important to assess whether their treatment plan adequately addresses their communication needs. Before medication is initiated, the need for increasing treatment goals by using augmentative or verbal forms of communication should be considered. Next, a careful assessment of the relative risk of medication use should be made. This chapter addresses specific indications for individual medications that are supported by research as well as points out when the research data are limited or inconclusive.

Some medications have strong, well-established evidence supporting their efficacy, while others have limited data resulting from shortcomings in research design or a paucity of studies. Often efficacy is reported based on a single clinical trial that has not been replicated through rigorous prospective, double-blind, controlled studies. Further, autism's inherent heterogeneity makes it a challenging condition to study. Many studies in this area use varying inclusion criteria and outcome measures, making it difficult to draw definitive conclusions about efficacy. These methodological limitations must be addressed before reliable conclusions can be made.

Reviews from clinical databases have shown that approximately 27% of all children who receive an autism diagnosis take at least one psychotropic medication; this statistic rises to 66% in the case of adolescents. Of the adolescents with co-occurring psychiatric diagnoses, the prevalence rate of those taking at least one medication rises to 80%. Those having lower intelligence quotients (IQs) and living in poverty are reported to have even higher psychopharmaceutical prescription rates. This disparity is most likely related to issues of limited or difficult access to specialists and other services, resulting in greater reliance on medication use by overtaxed clinicians caring for these children. The most common indications for psychopharmaceutical intervention are the presence of anxiety, depression, ADHD, irritability and disruptive behaviors (to one's functioning or others' space), compulsions, and repetitive behaviors.

The first step in evaluation for potential intervention is a review of symptoms. Most research studies use standardized measures such as the Aberrant Behavior Checklist (ABC) to define these indications. In the primary care setting, it is more likely that the clinician will carefully determine the presence of symptoms while assessing their severity, length, and frequency when considering a medication trial (refer to Chapter 9, Autism and Behavioral Challenges: Why They Occur and How to Approach Them, for a description of the **FINDS** acronym used to assess the effects of a behavior). This chapter reviews the clinical indications based on the child's manifesting symptoms and the available research data supporting the use of medications.

Treating Attention-Deficit/Hyperactivity Disorder

Coexisting ADHD occurs in 40% to 70% of children and adolescents on the autism spectrum. This secondary diagnosis in the context of autism is supported by the *Diagnostic and Statistical Manual of Mental Disorders, Fifth Edition, Text Revision.* As with any child being evaluated for an ADHD diagnosis, the collection of data from standardized questionnaires and classroom observations by multiple observers is imperative. Standardized behavioral scales (refer to Chapter 10, Diagnosing and Managing Co-Occurring Conditions, for more details) have not been validated with children on the spectrum for whom an ADHD diagnosis is being considered, but the use of these scales continues to be clinically useful when the diagnosis is being considered and the response to medication is being assessed. Educational supports and accommodations can be effective first-line interventions, including breaking tasks into steps, using visual supports, removing distractions, modifying demands and assignments, and providing access to regular check-ins with a teacher. If a child has started in a new classroom or their placement has been modified, a check-in must occur with the family and/or the school team before initiating medication, to be certain that supports remain constant and meet the needs detailed in the child's IEP.

When medication is initiated for children with both autism and ADHD, the same array of medications used in non-autistic children is considered. These are typically methylphenidate derivatives, amphetamine derivatives, and nonstimulant medications (clonidine, guanfacine, venlafaxine, viloxazine, and atomoxetine). Repeated studies demonstrate that children on the spectrum are more likely to experience adverse effects and they require the use of lower doses and slow titrations. Additionally, the response demonstrated is less robust in children with both autism and ADHD than in those with ADHD alone. This difference is likely caused by the complexities of overlapping symptoms, many of which are attributed to autism and are therefore less likely to respond to medications that target ADHD symptoms.

Data from the large double-blind, placebo-controlled crossover study performed by the Research Units on Pediatric Psychopharmacology (RUPP) Autism Network in 2005 were pivotal in supporting the use of psychostimulants in children with coexisting autism and ADHD. Hyperactivity was the symptom with the most noticeable improvement. Response to medication was defined as 49% improvement using the clinician-completed ABC Hyperactivity subscale and global (overall) scores as well as the Clinical Global Impressions–Improvement (CGI-I) scale. In this study, the response rate of autistic children with ADHD using twice-a-day fixed dosing of short-acting methylphenidate (0.125, 0.25, and 0.5 mg/kg/day) with a small afternoon dose was less robust than that of non-autistic children with ADHD (49% vs 77%). The adverse effects of social withdrawal and increased irritability were more commonly seen in autistic children with ADHD, causing 18% to discontinue medication. This is a higher rate of discontinuation than is observed among comparable non-autistic children. Other expected adverse effects, including insomnia, appetite suppression, and tics, are seen with similar rates in children on and not on the spectrum. At the outset, this study used fixed dosing, but later, when doses were titrated individually, adherence improved. Autistic children with ADHD responded optimally to doses a quarter to a half the dose used most often in non-autistic children.

There are several nonstimulant medications that have demonstrated efficacy in treating ADHD in children on the spectrum. α_2-Adrenergic agonists stimulate postsynaptic α_{2A} receptors in the prefrontal cortex, potentiating noradrenergic transmission. This action most likely mediates the therapeutic effects of guanfacine on working memory, attention, and behavioral control. These agents have demonstrated efficacy in small sample sizes of school-aged children with both autism and

ADHD. Efficacy was defined as demonstrating improvement on the CGI-I and was demonstrated in 50% of children in 2 studies, with the Hyperactivity subscale scores showing the most improvement. Drowsiness, irritability, and some nighttime awakenings were noted adverse effects that did not result in significant concern or discontinuation. No significant effect on blood pressure was documented.

The selective norepinephrine reuptake inhibitor atomoxetine has been shown to have mixed results in children and adolescents with both autism and ADHD as opposed to their non-autistic peers. In several randomized, double-blind, placebo-controlled trials, efficacy has been documented in Hyperactivity subscores, such as the CGI-I scale, but not in global improvement scores. Another study introduced a slow titration of atomoxetine, from 0.5 mg/kg up to 1.8 mg/kg, which showed more robust responses, with 67% of the study children demonstrating improvement. Atomoxetine is moderately well tolerated, with nausea, decreased appetite, and poor weight gain being the most interfering adverse effects. Additional reported adverse effects include fatigue and sleep interruption.

Venlafaxine, a serotonin-norepinephrine uptake inhibitor, has demonstrated promising global clinical improvement in a small retrospective clinical trial of autistic children with ADHD. In the study, 6 of 10 participants were felt to be responders, as defined by an improvement in CGI scores. The medication was well tolerated, but larger prospective studies are needed to substantiate this finding.

Viloxazine is a nonstimulant recently approved by the US Food and Drug Administration (FDA) for the treatment of ADHD in children 6 years and older. Its proposed mechanism of action is a combination of blocking the reuptake of norepinephrine and thereby increasing its availability, serotonin receptor modulation, and dopamine enhancement. A meta-analysis of its use in non-autistic children shows significant improvement on the ADHD Rating Scale-IV and the CGI-I scale when compared to that of the placebo group. The medication seems to be well tolerated, but only small samples of children with ADHD and autism have been studied.

In summary, there are solid research data to support the efficacious use of both stimulants and nonstimulants without causing harm in children with autism and ADHD, while the newer agents require replication in studies to confirm their efficacy.

Treating Anxiety

Specific and generalized anxiety are commonly seen in children on the autism spectrum. The combination of communication delays, RRBs, sensory vulnerabilities, and poor social skills places children on the spectrum at high risk for all forms of anxiety. Seemingly inconsequential triggers, such as a request to transition, walking by a noisy window, academic struggles, a demand to perform a challenging task, or internal sources of discomfort, may result in impairing anxiety for many children on the spectrum. This anxiety may manifest in nonspecific ways such as externalizing behavior, increased repetitive or stereotypical behavior, increased restricted behavior or resistance, or academic regression.

The Autism Treatment Network/Autism Intervention Research Network on Physical Health group developed practice parameters for autistic children with anxiety. If anxiety symptoms are present and of significant clinical concern, the recommendation is to treat any psychiatric or medical condition that may be causing or adding to the anxiety. The clinician must address any psychosocial stressors and ensure that educational and/or behavioral supports that are required to alleviate the anxiety are in place. If symptoms persist despite the introduction of accommodations and interventions, medications should be considered.

The selective serotonin reuptake inhibitor (SSRI) group of medications has the most rigorous data supporting its use. There is a lack of well-designed double-blind, placebo-controlled studies of autistic children with anxiety being treated with SSRIs, so the recommendations are predominantly extrapolated from the use of SSRIs in neurotypical children. To avoid the increased incidence of activation in autistic children being treated with SSRIs, a very slow titration up to the low starting doses should be initiated (**Table 13.1**). Use of a liquid preparation can be helpful in achieving this titration. Activation is expressed as increased activity, irritability, insomnia, or disinhibition. These symptoms tend to manifest as the drug is introduced or the dose is titrated upward. The activation may resolve if the dose is lowered or if the medication is discontinued. The child should be followed closely with monthly visits until the desired dose seems well tolerated. A family history of bipolar disorder places any individual at risk of precipitating manifestations of mania, and children and adolescents with such a family history would best be referred to specialists for management.

The FDA recommendations to support the use of the SSRIs are listed in **Table 13.1** and derived from research studies that document the safety profile in children. The availability of a liquid form of fluoxetine makes it a palatable choice for titration for younger children.

Table 13.1. Selective Serotonin Reuptake Inhibitor Medication Dosing

Medication[a]	Starting Dose, mg/day	Maximum Dose, mg/day	US Food and Drug Administration Approval Indications
Sertraline	12.5	200	OCD, panic disorders, social phobia, PTSD ≥6 y
Fluoxetine (available in liquid form)	2.5–5	60	OCD and panic disorders ≥7 y, MDD ≥8 y
Citalopram	2.5–5	40	
Escitalopram	1.25–2.5	20	GAD ≥6 y, MDD ≥12 y

Abbreviations: GAD, generalized anxiety disorder; MDD, major depressive disorder, OCD, obsessive-compulsive disorder; PTSD, posttraumatic stress disorder.

[a] Listed in order of frequency of use.

Treating Depression and Suicidal Ideation

Depression and suicidal ideation are prevalent among children on the autism spectrum. For the teenagers on the spectrum who have at least an average IQ, 35% of them (self-reported) and 75% of their parents (parent-reported) observed clinically significant levels of depressive symptoms. Girls were more likely to report symptoms of depression. Among autistic youth with depression, rates of suicidal ideation vary, with up to 32% reporting these thoughts. Diagnosing depression in children with lower verbal cognition can be challenging and requires a more comprehensive review of the child's performance across many settings and developmental domains. As was discussed in Chapter 10, Diagnosing and Managing Co-Occurring Conditions, depression and anxiety in a child on the spectrum may manifest in a nonspecific manner, such as academic regression, externalizing behaviors, regressive behavior, decline in self-care, or exacerbation of autism features. The prototypical manifestations seen in adults (change in appetite, sleep problems, or poor concentration) may not be obvious in children. As with all behavioral health concerns, evaluation for other causes of depression and use of psychotherapeutic intervention to best support the individual should be in place before any medication is introduced.

Pharmacological treatment of depression in autistic youth is based on research findings from non-autistic populations. Although the use of SSRIs appears to be safe, individuals on the spectrum are more susceptible to behavioral activation, irritability, and sleep disturbance from these medications. Dosing for SSRIs is the same as for anxiety and is reviewed in **Table 13.1**. Specialists support the use of low doses and slow titration if medication is necessary, as discussed in the previous section, Treating Anxiety.

Treating Irritability With Second-Generation Antipsychotic Medications

Irritability is expressed in children as repeated outbursts of anger, frustration, or distress. It is often manifested through acts of aggression directed toward oneself, another person, or a piece of property. Outbursts or aggressive behaviors tend to occur when feelings of distress or frustration exceed the individual's capacity to modulate their responses. Children on the autism spectrum tend to experience communication challenges and difficulties regulating their emotions, and when the expression of frustration is out of proportion to the trigger, the outbursts tend to negatively affect the child and the people living with or caring for them. When tantrums occur with high frequency (>2–3 times per day); are directed toward people, self, or property; occur outside the home; or occur with people other than the child's parents, the child is often brought to a medical care setting for evaluation and treatment. These behaviors can put others at risk, be destructive, negatively affect the child's ability to engage and learn, and represent a challenge that needs to be addressed. The pediatric clinician has an opportunity to intercede and refer these children for behavioral assessment and intervention before medication becomes necessary (refer to Chapter 9, Autism and Behavioral Challenges: Why They Occur and How to Approach Them). When medication management of irritability is being considered, most pediatric clinicians will rely on the specialists for consultation and support. It is not expected that the pediatric primary care clinician have the expertise to manage the use of antipsychotics independent of the specialist, but it is possible that with experience and consultation, the pediatric primary care clinician might initiate therapy independently.

Atypical antipsychotic medications (also referred to as *second-generation antipsychotics* [SGAs]) are used for irritability and disruptive behaviors that negatively affect the child and their family and should be considered only after all behavioral and educational interventions have been exhausted. Risperidone and aripiprazole are the only medications approved by the FDA for irritability in the context of autism. Risperidone is approved for ages 5 to 16 years; aripiprazole, for ages 6 to 16 years. Second-generation antipsychotic medications block postsynaptic dopamine and serotonin and they produce a lower risk for extrapyramidal adverse effects than the traditional first-generation agents (haloperidol or chlorpromazine). The RUPP Autism Network published a large, multisite placebo-controlled, double-blind study in 2002 that supports the use of risperidone for severe irritability in autistic children aged 5 to 7 years. Doses were individualized according to weight and tolerability, with a target daily dose of 2.5 mg for children weighing 20 to 45 kg and 3.5 mg for children weighing more than 45 kg.

The autistic children in the RUPP Autism Network study demonstrated a 56% reduction in irritability symptoms in comparison to a 14% reduction in the control group. In two-thirds of the children with a positive response to risperidone, the benefit was maintained at 6 months. Efficacy was also demonstrated for hyperactivity and stereotypy. Other open-label trials of risperidone have confirmed its efficacy but have also demonstrated frequent adverse effects, including short-term sedation, increased appetite, vomiting, excessive weight gain, and elevated prolactin levels. The larger RUPP Autism Network study included 101 children and adolescents aged 5 to 17 years and showed no occurrence of extrapyramidal effects. Adverse effects such as dizziness, fatigue, drooling, and constipation were short-term effects that did not result in discontinuation of treatment. The observed weight gain and increases in appetite varied in different studies. The RUPP Autism Network study reported 2.7-kg weight gain, whereas previous studies reported 5.6-kg weight gain, over the first 6 months of use, with weight gain leveling off thereafter.

Risperidone dosing is reviewed in **Table 13.2**. The advised dosage is 0.25 to 3 mg/day and is based on the efficacy demonstrated in the RUPP Autism Network study. The RUPP Autism Network found that the addition of a manualized parent training component augmented the efficacy of pharmacological intervention. Both

Table 13.2. Aripiprazole and Risperidone Dosing

Medication	Available Dosage, mg Tablets	Dosage Range, mg/day	Reduction in Irritability at 6 Months, %
Aripiprazole	2, 5, 10, 15, 20, 30	2–15	44–50
Risperidone	0.25, 0.5, 1, 2, 3, 4	0.25–3	56
Adverse effects: short-term sedation, increased appetite, excessive weight gain			

the medication and the medication plus parent training showed improvement that was statistically significant from that in the placebo group, but the combined group showed an advantage in improvement in the child's response to requests (defined as "noncompliance" in the study), irritability, and hyperactivity at 24 weeks of study. This finding further supports the recommendation that behavioral intervention always be included in the treatment plan.

Aripiprazole was later approved by the FDA for the treatment of irritability in autistic children and adolescents aged 6 to 17 years. Aripiprazole dosing is reviewed in **Table 13.2**. A large controlled study using fixed doses of 5, 10, and 15 mg of aripiprazole demonstrated strong efficacies of 43.8%, 47.8%, and 50.9%, respectively. Sedation was the main adverse effect and resolved in a median of 19 to 23 days. Weight gain was observed but was less than that seen with risperidone (1.3 kg at 8 weeks with aripiprazole vs 2.3 kg at 8 weeks with risperidone). At 1 year, the average weight gain was 6.3 kg, but weight gain plateaued over time. Serum lipid levels were also negatively affected over the first year of treatment. There are no long-term studies on the metabolic effects of antipsychotics, but clearly the added risk for metabolic syndrome is high and may be significant. No significant cardiac adverse effects were identified during the study period, thus negating the necessity of electrocardiographic screening. Of study participants, 14.5% discontinued drug treatment because of extrapyramidal symptoms (dystonia or involuntary movements or posturing, akathisia or restlessness, parkinsonism, and tardive dyskinesia). It was deduced that increasing the dosing of aripiprazole beyond 5 mg resulted in an increased risk for adverse effects, while the chance for increased drug efficacy was relatively small. When these medications are required, using the lowest dose possible, with slow and careful titration up to the target dose, is recommended to minimize adverse effects, while evaluating for efficacy after 4 to 6 weeks. As mentioned at the start of this chapter, Chapter 10, Diagnosing and Managing Co-Occurring Conditions, discusses the supports available to the primary care clinician in this process. Many states have free telephone consultations available with psychiatrists.

Alternative antipsychotics are not FDA approved for use in children on the spectrum, and research data are less favorable. Small open-label trials of olanzapine show conflicting efficacy as well as higher weight gain than seen with the 2 FDA-approved agents. Quetiapine has been found to have minimal efficacy and is poorly tolerated. Ziprasidone has limited data suggesting efficacy.

Anticonvulsants and mood stabilizers have shown mixed efficacy in treating irritability and disruptive behaviors and will be managed by specialists with expertise with these drugs. Divalproex sodium has been studied extensively with mixed results. Studies using divalproex have used varied inclusion criteria and have shown some success, although efficacy is not as significant as with the antipsychotics. Although divalproex is generally well tolerated, adverse effects, including behavioral activation, rash, sedation, nausea and vomiting, and weight gain, can be limiting factors. Further, it is required that serum medication levels and liver enzyme levels be monitored.

Two other anticonvulsants, lamotrigine and levetiracetam, showed limited results and conflicting results, respectively, in treating irritability alone. In small case studies, topiramate shows some promise, but similar to divalproex, it has a wide adverse effect profile that may limit its use. Lithium may have some efficacy as a rescue therapy for children who present with catatonia and also for treatment of those who have *SHANK* gene mutations (as seen in Phelan-McDermid syndrome). When treating irritability, anticonvulsants and mood stabilizers should be reserved for use by specialists in refractory cases.

Treating Restricted and Repetitive Behaviors

Restricted and repetitive behaviors are core features of autism that can interfere with functioning. There are few data to support the use of pharmacological agents to treat these and the other core features of autism directly. Selective serotonin reuptake inhibitors have minimal efficacy in treating stereotypical behaviors unless treating the underlying anxiety results in improvement. The use of omega-3 fatty acids or psychostimulants did not demonstrate efficacy with RRBs. Antipsychotic medications have demonstrated small but significant improvements for stereotypical behaviors, but their adverse effect profiles must be considered before using them for this indication. Buspirone may have some efficacy, but data require replication and further study before this medication can be recommended. Newer studies looking at treating core features of autism are discussed in the next section, Innovative Treatments. Currently, there is no demonstrated efficacy for psychopharmaceutical agents in the treatment of RRBs.

Innovative Treatments

More recent investigations have illuminated alterations in excitatory-inhibitory neurotransmitter pathways as possible mechanisms for the clinical presentations of autism. This research has studied the glutamate (excitatory) and γ-aminobutyric acid (GABA) (inhibitory) neurotransmitters in an attempt to target the core features of autism. These newer agents, discussed below, should be managed by specialists with expertise.

Memantine, an *N*-methyl-D-aspartate glutamate-type receptor antagonist, has mostly been studied to augment the effects of risperidone and other medications. Its use may result in improved clinical scale scores for irritability and language. When used alone, in a randomized, double-blind clinical trial of forty-two 8- to 17-year-old children and adolescents on the spectrum who had an IQ of 85 or greater, memantine was well tolerated. Children in the study demonstrated a 25% or greater improvement on informant-reported responses to the Social Responsiveness Scale, Second Edition (SRS-2), and a clinician-rated CGI-I subscale.

R-baclofen (arbaclofen) is a GABA-B agonist that has been used in people with multiple sclerosis as a muscle relaxant. Trials in autistic children with an average IQ of 56 demonstrate significant improvement in irritability, although not as robust as what was found in the RUPP Autism Network study for risperidone and aripiprazole (34% with arbaclofen vs 57% with risperidone). A phase 2 randomized, placebo-controlled trial including 150 autistic individuals aged 5 to 21 years demonstrated no difference between study participants and control group participants on the parent-rated ABC Social Withdrawal/Lethargy subscale. A secondary finding was improvement on the clinician-rated Clinical Global Impressions–Severity (CGI-S) scale and adaptive behaviors on the Vineland Adaptive Behavior Scales, Second Edition (Vineland-II), Socialization domain. There is a suggestion that arbaclofen may have the potential to improve some symptoms in children on the spectrum, but clearly further study is required, and no study has compared its efficacy head-to-head with that of an SGA agent. Use of arbaclofen resulted in affect lability in 11% of the participants and sedation in 9%.

The third medication postulated to treat the underlying pathophysiology of autism by reducing glutaminergic neurotransmission at synapses is *N*-acetylcysteine (NAC). NAC is a glutamate modulator that has been used to minimize liver damage during toxicity from acetaminophen overdose. It has also been used as an augmenting drug for a variety of psychiatric disorders (eg, bipolar disorders, schizophrenia). NAC is well tolerated, although the individual must take a large number of capsules to adequately reach an effective treatment dose. Additionally, it is considered a food supplement and is unavailable through pharmacies. Its use has demonstrated significant improvement in irritability and self-injurious behavior on the ABC similar to that achieved with atypical antipsychotics (57.4%), although no studies have compared NAC efficacy against efficacies of the SGA agents. The pooled results of a meta-analysis reveal significantly improved hyperactivity, irritability, and social awareness after an 8- to 12-week treatment trial using NAC. The target dose ranges from 50 to 400 mg daily. The recommended starting dose is 12.5 mg daily, with gradual weekly increases up to 50 mg, guided by ongoing assessments of the child's response to treatment.

The compound sulforaphane, an extract from broccoli, has received a great deal of attention in autism news and research. Sulforaphane has antioxidant effects allowing tissue to heal from stress and has been used in cancer prevention. A single randomized, double-blind, controlled study demonstrated statistically significant improvements in irritability and lethargy in adolescents and adults on the spectrum but not in stereotypy or hyperactivity. The SRS score improved and there was an overall improvement described in social interaction and verbal communication. This study requires replication with larger sample sizes and more controlled parameters. There is some indication that sulforaphane might be a helpful adjunctive treatment aimed at treating the underlying pathophysiology of autism. The effects were less robust than those observed with the antipsychotics and there are no long-term data.

Naltrexone, an opioid antagonist, has also been studied in children on the spectrum. Its potential therapeutic role is based on a theoretical model suggesting abnormalities in the opioid system associated with autism. Studies have demonstrated some efficacy, in which 8 of the 13 study children on the spectrum demonstrated a reduction in hyperactivity but not in any of the other core features of autism. Additionally, an older study from 2004 revealed that 47% of participants had a 50% or greater reduction in self-injurious behaviors. The use of naltrexone is limited by its bitter taste, and although adverse effects seem to be mild and transient, it is not regularly used in children on the spectrum.

Melatonin is an over-the-counter dietary supplement that has a good evidence basis for its use in the context of sleep latency insomnia in children on the spectrum. Trials have reported a positive effect on sleep physiology without significant associated adverse effects. The use of melatonin is discussed in more detail in Chapter 12, Insomnia: Identification and Interventions.

Complementary and Alternative Treatments

The use of complementary (in addition to conventional medical approaches) and alternative (in lieu of traditional medical approaches) treatments is very common in the United States. According to the 2007 National Health Interview Survey, 38% of adults and 11.8% of children use at least one form of complementary and alternative medicine (CAM). Within the context of autism, families report use in 28% to 75% of children on the spectrum. Families that tend to use complementary treatments often use medical treatments in general and tend to use these interventions in addition to more conventional practices.

The most common types of CAM are natural products (up to 54%) such as herbs, vitamins, and probiotics; special diets (up to 33%); and mind and body practices (up to 30%). Most families choose to use these products and practices to treat coexisting conditions in children on the spectrum, such as hyperactivity, irritability, GI symptoms, seizures, sleep disruption, and sensory vulnerabilities. Most individuals and families that use CAM will implement more than one agent or practice and tend to obtain information about CAM from sources other than their primary care clinicians.

It is important for clinicians to include information about the use of complementary treatments in the care they provide for families of children on the spectrum. Many families may underreport their use of CAM treatments; thus, families should be directly asked about their practices. This approach presents an opportunity for the pediatric primary care clinician to partner with the family. By entering into this partnership, the clinician will learn about the family's understanding of clinical presentations and how they approach and prioritize treatments and personal resources. The recommendations for the use of CAM often originate from lay sources rather than professional review and can involve expense, attention focused away from more effective interventions, and risk for negative side effects and potential drug interactions. The pediatric primary care clinician has an opportunity to guide families as they make decisions that may affect the entire family as well as the child.

The research data on the use of CAM are complicated, and few of the studies are believed to have methodology sufficient to make strong recommendations. Study samples are small and heterogenous, and outcome measures not only are varied but often are reliant on parents, teachers, or other observers who are not blinded to the treatment, which may create bias. There are an exhaustive number of these agents under investigation, and this section reviews those most frequently used. There are some reports that suggest possible positive responses, but none are related to the core features of autism.

Equine therapy has shown positive improvements on behavioral scales in studies that contain methodological weaknesses likely leading to biased reporting. The positive effects reported with music therapy have unclear clinical relevance. Initial small clinical trials demonstrated some efficacy in emotional recognition and eye gaze, but larger follow-up studies using more rigorous methodology did not support efficacy.

Elimination diets are strongly recommended for children on the spectrum by many autism groups but not by the medical community. The research on the use of a gluten-free/casein-free diet demonstrated positive effects when parents reported the outcome, with no effect demonstrated when the study was administered in a controlled, double-blind trial. The concern for a suspected placebo effect is discussed in Chapter 11, Gastrointestinal Symptoms and Feeding Challenges.

Other more invasive therapies have demonstrated conflicting outcomes and have not resulted in recommendations for their use by the medical community. These therapies target the theory of immune dysfunction as a cause of autism. Results have been inconsistent and inconclusive. One such therapy is hyperbaric oxygen therapy, which is rarely recommended and clearly has a large financial and logistical burden associated with its use.

Stem cell transplant is another biomedical therapy studied to treat the inflammatory processes and immune dysfunction thought to be associated with autism.

Clinical trials using stem cell transplant in children on the spectrum who had not responded to conventional therapies have been effective in reducing scores on autism rating scales without causing significant negative side effects. Meta-analyses report these global improvements of statistical significance, but concern about small sample size and limited methodology in phase 1 studies suggests that the findings require validation. The single phase 2 study performed at Duke University, the Acceptance and Commitment Therapy study, was a randomized, double-blind, controlled crossover study assessing the efficacy of autologous and allogenic cord blood infusions in 180 children aged 2 to 7 years with documented autism. Although the infusion was found to be safe and without significant adverse events, there was no global improvement seen in core autism features that were interfering with functioning or in socialization. A subgroup with IQ scores greater than 70 were found to have improved communication scores only. No conclusion was drawn that stem cell infusion is an effective treatment as studied.

Neurofeedback is a technique used to train participants to self-regulate electroencephalographic (EEG) brain activity and improve attention, emotional regulation, and cognitive function. The individual receives auditory or video feedback as they are engaged in activity. Given that atypical EEG patterns are commonly seen in those on the spectrum, and there is concern for imbalance of the excitatory and inhibitory mechanisms in the brain, neurofeedback may be a mechanism for encouraging remodeling of neural circuits within the context of autism. Neurofeedback is thought to have some therapeutic potential. Studies have documented its feasibility in children on the spectrum with different cognitive potentials. There was a single clinical trial with no control group that demonstrated the positive effect of a 10-week neurofeedback trial on executive functioning, processing speed, and working memory on a small group of autistic children and adolescents aged 7 to 17 years. This study requires validation. Similar well-designed studies in children with ADHD alone do not consistently demonstrate efficacy on cognitive function. Neurofeedback may prove to be an adjunctive tool for children with these types of developmental profiles.

Recent interest in a possible connection between the gut microbiome and autism has motivated researchers to assess the therapeutic value of prebiotics (indigestible starches that stimulate bacterial growth), probiotics (living microbes that support a healthy gut), and fecal transplant (the transfer of healthy fecal matter from a donor to a recipient). The working hypothesis is that dysbiosis (alterations in the variety of microbes in the gut) could be related to the differences in brain function observed in those on the spectrum. Attempts at performing reviews and a meta-analysis of the research available point out the many methodological weaknesses of the literature, limiting the ability to draw conclusions about the therapeutic value of these interventions.

Most therapies, including the use of vitamins and supplements, carry the potential for negative side effects. While taking vitamins at the recommended daily allowance is generally considered safe, high-dose supplementation of nutrients such as magnesium and vitamin B_6 has been explored in individuals on the spectrum. Studies have indicated a risk for toxicity with these higher doses. Additionally, there is limited evidence to support the efficacy of these treatments. Well-designed studies have shown no clear benefits from the use of vitamins, herbal products, probiotics, auditory integration therapy, acupuncture, craniosacral manipulation, antifungal or antibiotic treatments of bacterial overgrowth, intravenous immunoglobulins, digestive enzymes, or secretin.

Chelation therapy, which has been periodically popular in treating autism, is based on the unproven theory of heavy metal accumulation in those on the spectrum. Chelation has not only failed to demonstrate effectiveness in addressing concerns around autism but also carries significant risks and potential toxicity. A case of death attributed to chelation therapy has led to a sharp decline in its use. These concerns underscore the importance of clinicians being aware of their patients' use of CAM therapies.

The research on cannabinoids is similarly inconclusive. Most of the studies are retrospective gatherings of data on global clinical improvement, aberrant behaviors, sleep, hyperactivity, and seizures. These indicate some improvement when cannabinoids of varying combinations and doses of cannabidiol and tetrahydrocannabinol are administered. There is no ability to extrapolate these results to clinical use because of the many shortcomings in methodology. The adverse effects reported are equally variable and concerning, with one study documenting that 51% of participants had at least one significant adverse effect. In summary, results are not yet of clinical relevance from cannabinoid administration, none of these cannabinoid substances are FDA approved for children on the spectrum, and many have the potential for significant adverse effects.

Although there are novel and encouraging treatment modalities used in individuals on the spectrum, currently the variable quality of research methodologies limits the ability to recommend these interventions. Often parents read reports based on small clinical trials that have not been replicated through larger prospective and well-designed studies with long-term data. Parents may obtain information from other parents or the internet without an appreciation for the limitations of these reports. Families anxious to achieve a positive effect on their child's course may be willing to make sacrifices that distract from the evidence-based treatment and may therefore adversely affect the long-term well-being of the entire family. It is incumbent on the clinician to ask regularly about CAM use and review the criteria necessary for accurate interpretation of recommendations to be certain there is no harm being done by their use. Parents seeking a cure or an alleviation of the challenges that may result from their child's autism may be more likely to try agents without solid efficacy or safety profiles. A careful discussion of a family's belief system and an open dialogue of the risks and benefits of alternative treatments are essential as clinicians work to ensure optimal outcomes while keeping the child safe.

CASE VIGNETTE: CONCLUSION

Eva returns with her parents for an appointment. She is very active and explores the room, touching many objects and talking constantly, and she becomes upset when the primary care clinician attempts to examine her. Both the clinician and the parents attempt to reassure Eva and explain what is going to happen, but she continues to become agitated and upset and goes to the door, asking to leave. When her parents do not respond, Eva becomes more upset and begins to bang on the door and grab her mother. She cannot be redirected or comforted and eventually begins to hit her mother and hit her own head while asking repeatedly to go home. The clinician attempts a brief physical examination and performs a review of systems to rule out possible coexisting medical conditions. The appointment ends and a follow-up appointment is made with the parents alone.

The following areas of concern and aspects of care are identified:

- Irritability and disruptive behaviors: Eva has increasingly more severe, more frequent, and more interfering irritability and behavioral outbursts that need to be better understood. She is having daily outbursts that are challenging to resolve. It is unclear whether there are specific triggers for her behavior, and her behavioral responses indicate that the daily demands placed on her outstrip her ability to regulate her emotions. She has few coping skills. A review of stressors, including family dynamics, financial needs, and exposures to violence or loss, as well as supports available to the family, reveals no significant contributors. There is no concern raised for contributing medical conditions, and primary irritability is approached in the following manner with her treatment team and the school:
  - Functional behavioral assessment (FBA) (refer to Chapter 9, Autism and Behavioral Challenges: Why They Occur and How to Approach Them): It is determined that an FBA is needed to collect more information about the antecedents and consequences of Eva's behaviors. It is evident that there is anxiety, that there is a fair amount of difficulty in flexibility, and that her behaviors are serving a function to allow her to avoid nonpreferred demands. The family is referred for work with a behavioral specialist to perform the FBA and determine what new treatment goals and behavioral interventions are required to ensure progress.
  - Recognizing difficulty in cognitive flexibility and teaching flexibility: These items will need to be integrated into Eva's educational goals. Teaching her the concept of flexibility and providing concrete examples of how she can practice flexibility, while providing incentives for her efforts, will be an important part of her therapy inside and outside of school.
  - Review of medical history and examination for possible medical contributors: It is determined that there is no evidence of GI distress, dental pain, pruritus, allergies, sinus pressure, headache, medication adverse effects, or insomnia contributing to her irritability (refer to Box 9.4 in Chapter 9, Autism and Behavioral Challenges: Why They Occur and How to Approach Them). Additionally, the primary care clinician performs a review for possible stressors or social drivers of health, which is negative for contributors (refer to Box 9.5 in Chapter 9).

Continued on next page

- Communication: Eva struggles to use her language to communicate when she is stressed, is unhappy, or needs help. She will work with a team composed of a therapist (speech pathologist, occupational therapist, or educator) to put a program together through which they can identify the triggers for her tantrums and teach her strategies to regulate her emotional responses: she will work on using a form of communication to ask for help, identifying when she is upset, and using strategies for self-regulation. These may include doing deep breathing, taking a break, or using sensory tools.
- Accommodations: An assessment will determine which accommodations are likely to help Eva understand expectations and routines. Consideration of using visual schedules, breaking down demands into small chunks, and providing regular check-ins with an adult may be helpful. A visual schedule for visiting the doctor will be suggested.
- Medication use: After the school and Eva's behavioral team have consulted, Eva returns with her parents to discuss the use of medication for anxiety and irritability. The pediatric primary care clinician reviews with Eva's parents the risks and benefits of both SSRIs and antipsychotics, and questions are answered. The primary care clinician and parents decide to attempt treatment of Eva's anxiety with fluoxetine first. Unfortunately, despite a slow titration, Eva becomes quickly activated by the starting dose, with increased irritability, trouble settling at bedtime, and hyperactivity. This medication is discontinued. The clinician next recommends a trial of aripiprazole, after collecting baseline blood glucose and fasting lipid levels. The family is in agreement with beginning this medication. Her family is given a prescription for 2-mg tablets and they are told that Eva should take half of a tablet daily for the first month. Eva's parents are told to expect some somnolence initially, so it is recommended that she take her medication in the evenings.

  Eva returns within 1 month with mild improvement and without adverse effects. Her dose is then gradually increased at each visit in 1-mg increments over the next 3 months to a final dose of 5 mg daily. At this point, Eva's parents and teachers note tremendous improvement in her irritability and disruptive behaviors. She seems less hyperactive as well, with improved ability to settle at night. Eva's parents report that her appetite is notably increased and they have had to lock up snack foods or she will eat almost continually. Her weight has increased 5 lb since beginning the medication, and although her parents inquire about increasing the dose further, her primary care clinician encourages them to monitor her responses to the behavioral interventions put into place and her weight gain before a decision is made to further increase her dose. In the interim, a plan is introduced to increase exercise and attention to her nutritional and caloric intake and consider consultation with a nutritionist. Every 6 months, her primary care clinician orders a fasting lipid profile, blood glucose test, and blood pressure measurement and reviews her weight, height, and body mass index, as well as any neurological side effects.

This chapter has provided guidance for primary care clinicians to best understand how medication is used in children and adolescents on the autism spectrum. In the clinical setting, pediatric primary care clinicians should use clinical judgment individualized to each patient to make specific medication decisions and weigh risk-benefit profiles. Consideration of whether the child is able to swallow a pill, is able to chew a chewable, or requires a tasteless liquid is necessary in the decision-making as well. If there is concern about the child's weight gain or sleep onset, that may influence the choice of medications. If the child has emotional reactivity or dysregulation in the face of ADHD, the first line of treatment may be using a nonstimulant rather than a stimulant that may exacerbate these symptoms. In other children, the clinician will need to decide which clinical feature is primary and should therefore be treated first by consulting with the child's team of specialists. There are likely to be situations in which medications used for one indication are layered on medications used for an additional indication. There are ample resources to support the use of these medications, and such resources are frequently updated and available for guidance. These have been referenced earlier in the chapter and are noted again in the next section, Clinical Pearls. Each clinician will develop a comfort level in managing their patients' care over time, by obtaining feedback through specialist consultations and clinical experience.

Medication management should be viewed as an additional tool available to the primary care clinician who has assumed the role of case management for the autistic child and their family. It is a tool that should be integrated into the multidisciplinary educational and behavioral treatments used for co-occurring conditions and support optimal developmental progress.

Clinical Pearls

Highlights about the use of medication in treating the coexisting conditions of autism are as follows:

- ADHD
  - The stimulants (methylphenidate and amphetamine derivatives) are first-line therapeutic choices and are most effective and available in either a short- or long-acting form. For more information, refer to the Northwell Health ADHD Medication Guide (https://adhdmedicationguide.com) and *Pediatric Psychopharmacology for Primary Care,* 4th Edition, published by the AAP. Clinicians should start with low doses and titrate slowly. Clinicians should aim to target a quarter to a half the dose used in neurotypical youth.
  - The nonstimulants (α_2-adrenergic agonists, guanfacine and clonidine, and the SSRI atomoxetine) are safe and effective and can be used alone or in addition to a stimulant.
  - Children on the autism spectrum are more sensitive to adverse effects, and their response is less robust than in neurotypical youth.

Continued on next page

- Anxiety and/or depression
  - Efficacy and safety of SSRI use have been documented in neurotypical youth and are extrapolated to those on the spectrum.
  - Fluoxetine, sertraline, citalopram, and escitalopram are SSRIs that are used as first-line interventions.
  - Youth on the spectrum are at risk for activation (increased activity, irritability, and/or insomnia) when beginning an SSRI or as doses are increased. They will need close follow-up at these times.
  - Clinicians should titrate dosing very slowly. Use of a liquid preparation may make titration more easily achievable.
  - Many children and adolescents on the spectrum have positive clinical responses to low doses of SSRIs (eg, 10 mg of fluoxetine or 25 mg of sertraline).
- Irritability, self-injurious behavior, and/or aggression
  - The SGAs, aripiprazole and risperidone, are FDA approved for this indication.
  - These medications are most effective when used in conjunction with behavioral therapies.
  - The adverse effect profiles of SGAs, including excessive weight gain, the potential for metabolic effect, and/or initial somnolence, which tends to resolve, must be considered and discussed.
- Restricted and repetitive behaviors
  - Medications demonstrate little efficacy.
  - The only medications that are associated with reduced RRBs are antipsychotic medications, but their risk profiles limit their use for this indication.

References

Accordino RE, Kidd C, Politte LC, Henry CA, McDougle CJ. Psychopharmacological interventions in autism spectrum disorder. *Expert Opin Pharmacother.* 2016;17(7):937–952 PMID: 26891879 doi: 10.1517/14656566.2016.1154536

Alsayouf HA, Alsarhan O, Khreisat W, Daoud A. Atomoxetine treatment of attention deficit/hyperactivity disorder symptoms in 3–6-year-old children with autism spectrum disorder: a retrospective cohort study. *Children (Basel).* 2024;11(2):163 PMID: 38397275 doi: 10.3390/children11020163

Chandrasekhar T, Sikich L. Challenges in the diagnosis and treatment of depression in autism spectrum disorders across the lifespan. *Dialogues Clin Neurosci.* 2015;17(2):219–227 PMID: 26246795 doi: 10.31887/DCNS.2015.17.2/tchandrasekhar

Dawson G, Sun JM, Baker J, et al. A phase II randomized clinical trial of the safety and efficacy of intravenous umbilical cord blood infusion for treatment of children with autism spectrum disorder. *J Pediatr.* 2020;222:164–173.e5 PMID: 32444220 doi: 10.1016/j.jpeds.2020.03.011

Fung LK, Mahajan R, Nozzolillo A, et al. Pharmacologic treatment of severe irritability and problem behaviors in autism: a systematic review and meta-analysis. *Pediatrics.* 2016;137(suppl 2):S124–S135 PMID: 26908468 doi: 10.1542/peds.2015-2851K

Fusar-Poli L, Cavone V, Tinacci S, et al. Cannabinoids for people with ASD: a systematic review of published and ongoing studies. *Brain Sci.* 2020;10(9):572 PMID: 32825313 doi: 10.3390/brainsci10090572

Gegelashvili M. Autism and depression. *Georgian Med News.* 2019;(292–293):54–56 PMID: 31560663

Goel R, Hong JS, Findling RL, Ji NY. An update on pharmacotherapy of autism spectrum disorder in children and adolescents. *Int Rev Psychiatry.* 2018;30(1):78–95 PMID: 29693461 doi: 10.1080/09540261.2018.1458706

Greenhill LL, Swanson JM, Vitiello B, et al. Impairment and deportment responses to different methylphenidate doses in children with ADHD: the MTA titration trial. *J Am Acad Child Adolesc Psychiatry.* 2001;40(2):180–187 PMID: 11211366 doi: 10.1097/00004583-200102000-00012

Handen BL, Aman MG, Arnold LE, et al. Atomoxetine, parent training, and their combination in children with autism spectrum disorder and attention-deficit/hyperactivity disorder. *J Am Acad Child Adolesc Psychiatry.* 2015;54(11):905–915 PMID: 26506581 doi: 10.1016/j.jaac.2015.08.013

Handen BL, Sahl R, Hardan AY. Guanfacine in children with autism and/or intellectual disabilities. *J Dev Behav Pediatr.* 2008;29(4):303–308 PMID: 18552703 doi: 10.1097/DBP.0b013e3181739b9d

Harfterkamp M, van de Loo-Neus G, Minderaa RB, et al. A randomized double-blind study of atomoxetine versus placebo for attention-deficit/hyperactivity disorder symptoms in children with autism spectrum disorder. *J Am Acad Child Adolesc Psychiatry.* 2012;51(7):733–741 PMID: 22721596 doi: 10.1016/j.jaac.2012.04.011

Hasslinger J, Jonsson U, Bölte S. Immediate and sustained effects of neurofeedback and working memory training on cognitive functions in children and adolescents with ADHD: a multi-arm pragmatic randomized controlled trial. *J Atten Disord.* 2022;26(11):1492–1506 PMID: 35034510 doi: 10.1177/10870547211063645

Hollander E, Kaplan A, Cartwright C, Reichman D. Venlafaxine in children, adolescents, and young adults with autism spectrum disorders: an open retrospective clinical report. *J Child Neurol.* 2000;15(2):132–135 PMID: 10695900 doi: 10.1177/088307380001500214

Hyman SL, Levy SE, Myers SM, et al; American Academy of Pediatrics Council on Children With Disabilities and Section on Developmental and Behavioral Pediatrics. Identification, evaluation, and management of children with autism spectrum disorder. *Pediatrics.* 2020;145(1):e20193447 PMID: 31843864 doi: 10.1542/peds.2019-3447

Joshi G, Gönenc A, DiSalvo M, et al. Memantine to treat social impairment in youths with autism spectrum disorder: a randomized clinical trial. *JAMA Netw Open.* 2025;8(10):e2534927 PMID: 41032298 doi: 10.1001/jamanetworkopen.2025.34927

Lee TM, Lee KM, Lee CY, Lee HC, Tam KW, Loh EW. Effectiveness of *N*-acetylcysteine in autism spectrum disorders: a meta-analysis of randomized controlled trials. *Aust N Z J Psychiatry.* 2021;55(2):196–206 PMID: 32900213 doi: 10.1177/0004867420952540

Levy SE, Hyman SL. Complementary and alternative medicine treatments for children with autism spectrum disorders. *Child Adolesc Psychiatr Clin N Am.* 2015;24(1):117–143 PMID: 25455579 doi: 10.1016/j.chc.2014.09.004

Martínez-González AE, Andreo-Martínez P. Prebiotics, probiotics and fecal microbiota transplantation in autism: a systematic review. *Rev Psiquiatr Salud Ment (Engl Ed).* 2020;13(3):150–164 PMID: 32684346 doi: 10.1016/j.rpsm.2020.06.002

McCracken JT, McGough J, Shah B, et al; Research Units on Pediatric Psychopharmacology Autism Network. Risperidone in children with autism and serious behavioral problems. *N Engl J Med.* 2002;347(5):314–321 PMID: 12151468 doi: 10.1056/NEJMoa013171

Qu J, Liu Z, Li L, et al. Efficacy and safety of stem cell therapy in children with autism spectrum disorders: a systematic review and meta-analysis. *Front Pediatr.* 2022;10:897398 PMID: 35601435 doi: 10.3389/fped.2022.897398

Research Units on Pediatric Psychopharmacology Autism Network. Randomized, controlled, crossover trial of methylphenidate in pervasive developmental disorders with hyperactivity. *Arch Gen Psychiatry.* 2005;62(11):1266–1274 PMID: 16275814 doi: 10.1001/archpsyc.62.11.1266

Salazar F, Baird G, Chandler S, et al. Co-occurring psychiatric disorders in preschool and elementary school-aged children with autism spectrum disorder. *J Autism Dev Disord.* 2015;45(8):2283–2294 PMID: 25737019 doi: 10.1007/s10803-015-2361-5

Saleem S, Habib SH. Neurofeedback recuperates cognitive functions in children with autism spectrum disorders (ASD). *J Autism Dev Disord.* 2024;54(8):2891–2901 PMID: 37314667 doi: 10.1007/s10803-023-06037-z

Sampedro Baena L, Fuente GAC, Martos-Cabrera MB, et al. Effects of neurofeedback in children with attention-deficit/hyperactivity disorder: a systematic review. *J Clin Med.* 2021;10(17):3797 PMID: 34501246 doi: 10.3390/jcm10173797

Sanchack KE, Thomas CA. Autism spectrum disorder: primary care principles. *Am Fam Physician.* 2016;94(12):972–979 PMID: 28075089

Scahill L, McCracken JT, King BH, et al; Research Units on Pediatric Psychopharmacology Autism Network. Extended-release guanfacine for hyperactivity in children with autism spectrum disorder. *Am J Psychiatry.* 2015;172(12):1197–1206 PMID: 26315981 doi: 10.1176/appi.ajp.2015.15010055

Sikich L, Kolevzon A, King BH, et al. Intranasal oxytocin in children and adolescents with autism spectrum disorder. *N Engl J Med.* 2021;385(16):1462–1473 PMID: 34644471 doi: 10.1056/NEJMoa2103583

Singh K, Connors SL, Macklin EA, et al. Sulforaphane treatment of autism spectrum disorder (ASD). *Proc Natl Acad Sci USA.* 2014;111(43):15550–15555 PMID: 25313065 doi: 10.1073/pnas.1416940111

Symons FJ, Thompson A, Rodriguez MC. Self-injurious behavior and the efficacy of naltrexone treatment: a quantitative synthesis. *Ment Retard Dev Disabil Res Rev.* 2004;10(3):193–200 PMID: 15611982 doi: 10.1002/mrdd.20031

Vasa RA, Mazurek MO, Mahajan R, et al. Assessment and treatment of anxiety in youth with autism spectrum disorders. *Pediatrics.* 2016;137(suppl 2):S115–S123 PMID: 26908467 doi: 10.1542/peds.2015-2851J

Veenstra-VanderWeele J, Cook EH, King BH, et al. Arbaclofen in children and adolescents with autism spectrum disorder: a randomized, controlled, phase 2 trial. *Neuropsychopharmacology.* 2017;42(7):1390–1398 PMID: 27748740 doi: 10.1038/npp.2016.237

Villarreal-Martínez L, González-Martínez G, Sáenz-Flores M, et al. Stem cell therapy in the treatment of patients with autism spectrum disorder: a systematic review and meta-analysis. *Stem Cell Rev Rep.* 2022;18(1):155–164 PMID: 34515938 doi: 10.1007/s12015-021-10257-0

Wijnhoven LA, Niels-Kessels H, Creemers DH, Vermulst AA, Otten R, Engels RC. Prevalence of comorbid depressive symptoms and suicidal ideation in children with autism spectrum disorder and elevated anxiety symptoms. *J Child Adolesc Ment Health.* 2019;31(1):77–84 PMID: 31109252 doi: 10.2989/17280583.2019.1608830

Wood JJ, Kendall PC, Wood KS, et al. Cognitive behavioral treatments for anxiety in children with autism spectrum disorder: a randomized clinical trial. *JAMA Psychiatry.* 2020;77(5):474–483 PMID: 31755906 doi: 10.1001/jamapsychiatry.2019.4160

Yu CL, Kao YC, Thompson T, et al. Response trajectories and temporal trends of viloxazine treatment for young people with ADHD: a meta-analysis. *JAMA Netw Open.* 2024;7(11):e2445885 PMID: 39560942 doi: 10.1001/jamanetworkopen.2024.45885

Zhou MS, Nasir M, Farhat LC, Kook M, Artukoglu BB, Bloch MH. Meta-analysis: pharmacologic treatment of restricted and repetitive behaviors in autism spectrum disorders. *J Am Acad Child Adolesc Psychiatry.* 2021;60(1):35–45 PMID: 32387445 doi: 10.1016/j.jaac.2020.03.007

CHAPTER

14

Working With Special Education Services: A Primer

CASE VIGNETTE

Evan is a rising second grader who received autism services in kindergarten and first grade within a special education classroom. He received an autism diagnosis at age 2 years and intensive applied behavior analysis services during the preschool years. When he entered kindergarten, his communication skills were felt to be age appropriate and his individualized education program (IEP) focused on peer social engagement and flexibility. Evan demonstrated strengths in his early academic skills. He was reported to be reading grade-level books, to have a strong memory for recall, to be able to answer questions about content he read, and to enjoy performing simple addition and subtraction. At the end of first grade, Evan's teachers felt he was performing at grade level across the board. He was due for his triannual reevaluation, but the IEP team believed that he no longer qualified for special education services and that a reevaluation was no longer necessary. Evan and a parent come to the primary care clinician's office for Evan's health supervision appointment to discuss this recommendation.

In the United States, all children with demonstrated delays significantly affecting their communication; their physical, cognitive, social, and emotional development; and/or their adaptive skills are eligible for special education services. Federal mandates determine the rights of individuals with such delays, which have risen to the level of disabilities, but the application of these laws varies greatly from one county or state to another. At a time when private resources may be limited, when wait lists to see specialists are long, and when insurance reimbursement is limited, the pediatric primary care clinician is the accessible professional to assist parents in understanding their rights under the law or to refer them to work with special education advocates, attorneys, or nonprofit organizations that assist with advocacy within the school. This chapter is meant to serve as a resource and reference for the pediatric primary care clinician to learn about advocacy for the child with a disability or neurodivergence who is receiving special education services. This chapter reviews applicable special education laws and describes how the pediatric primary care clinician can learn about helping families navigate the special education system and the resources within their community.

A Brief History of Special Education Law

The US Supreme Court became involved in the right of all children, regardless of race, to obtain an education in 1954 in *Brown v Board of Education* and determined that "the opportunity of an education...is a right which must be made available to all on equal terms." Public Law No. 94-142 extended this right to all children with disabilities in 1972. The Education for All Handicapped Children Act was enacted in 1975. At that time, studies determined that less than half of children with disabilities were receiving an appropriate education and many were deprived of the opportunity to become educated and prepared to live independently. This law was intended to provide educational services to all children who qualified. It was not until 1990 that autism was listed as a disability that qualified children for special education services. In 2004, the Individuals with Disabilities Education Act (IDEA) refined these rights. It articulated that special education services must include the following components:

- Expectations for age-appropriate academic standards
- Access to the general education curriculum in a general education setting
- Preparation for life skills (activities of daily living [ADLs])
- Ensured parental participation in the special education process
- Training of high-quality teachers
- Use of evidence-based curricula and teaching strategies
- Application of classroom accommodations
- Access to assistive technology and other adaptive equipment

In IDEA §1400(d), it became law that the child meeting criteria for special education has "available to them a free appropriate public education that emphasizes special education and related services designed to meet their unique needs and prepare them for further education, employment, and independent living." Additionally, the law ensures that "the rights of children with disabilities and parents of such children are protected." Ideally, this part of the law should be familiar to the pediatric primary care clinician and can be used when advocating for each child found to be eligible for special education services. The services specified in an individualized family service plan (IFSP) or IEP should meet the needs of the child and prepare them to complete their education and to live independently. The special education process and the components of the IFSP and the IEP are reviewed in this chapter.

The Evaluation

The pediatric primary care clinician should be familiar with the referral process for early intervention (EI) services and evaluation for special education within their jurisdictions. Observations, screenings, and diagnostic work performed by the clinician are relevant to the screening process performed by EI/special education teams and should be shared with the team. Parents benefit from involvement of the clinician in the referral process, in the EI evaluation, and, most importantly, in the determination of appropriate educational services, including placement and monitoring of progress over time.

Parents, school staff, and state or local agencies may request an initial screening and evaluation by EI or special education service professionals when concern has been identified for delays in development. Parents may be unaware of this right, and this possibility presents another opportunity for the pediatric primary care clinician to advocate for the early introduction of evaluations and services. For Part C of IDEA, which outlines EI services for children 0 to 3 years of age, the family should contact their local EI/Child Find services for screening. For special education services for children older than 3 years, the parent will submit a written request for evaluation to their child's elementary school (refer to Appendix G, Sample Letter to Request Evaluation for Special Education Services). By law, this initial evaluation and determination of eligibility must be completed within a specified number days of the request, usually between 45 and 60 days. (These timelines may vary depending on the services being requested and the rules of the jurisdiction.) If this evaluation is initiated by someone other than a parent, parental consent is required for the evaluation to proceed. If the child meets criteria for evaluation after an initial screening, the law does not specify the content of the evaluation. The parent may identify areas of concern and advocate for specific areas of testing. The data provided by the testing serve to guide the development of the IFSP/IEP, if the child is determined to be eligible for services. It is therefore very important that this evaluation cover all relevant areas of the child's development. When meeting eligibility for services, the child 0 to 3 years of age will receive an IFSP and the services will be provided in the child's natural environment. The child older than 3 years will receive an IEP and the services will be school based. The IFSP focuses on skills that affect the child in the home or child care setting, whereas the IEP addresses the effect of school-based services on the child's participation in the classroom.

The IFSP and the IEP should be thought of as legal documents describing the child's rights within the public school setting. If some developmental domains are not evaluated and relevant disabilities not documented, the child has no binding right to receive services in these areas. The pediatric primary care clinician should review the process with the parent and aid the parent in making a list of all developmental domains that are relevant to autism and their particular child. With the support of the primary care clinician, the parent can be guided to make specific requests that ensure the evaluation is broad based and comprehensive, uses accurate tools, and is performed by relevant professionals.

The school evaluation team is composed of a special educator, a school psychologist, the general education teacher, and an administrator. On request, speech and occupational therapists, deaf and hard of hearing specialists, behavioral specialists, and outside specialists can be included. Ideally, the evaluation of the child with a possible or definitive diagnosis of autism should include the following information:

- Psychological data, including an intelligence quotient (IQ) or developmental quotient (DQ) based on findings from administered testing and not solely on responses from parent questionnaires.
- Findings from educational testing of the present levels of performance in all academic/developmental areas.
- Measure of adaptive functioning, typically using the Vineland Adaptive Behavior Scales (Vineland) or the Adaptive Behavior Assessment System (ABAS).
- Complete speech assessment, including some measure of language pragmatics or a qualitative language sampling of conversational abilities.
- Occupational therapy assessment of fine motor skills, motor coordination, and sensory processing.
- Responses from parent and teacher questionnaires addressing core features of autism, which may include the Autism Spectrum Rating Scales (ASRS), the Social Responsiveness Scale (SRS), and/or a broad behavioral screening for internalizing and externalizing behaviors (eg, the Child Behavior Checklist [CBCL], the Behavior Assessment System for Children [BASC], the Conners Comprehensive Behavior Rating Scales [Conners CBRS]).
- Descriptions of behavioral observations from a structured classroom activity, a time of transition, and/or a period of unstructured peer play. These may provide valuable information about the child's behavior responding to academic demands, social interaction, play, attention to tasks, persistence with tasks, transitions, and disruptive behaviors (to one's functioning or others' space).

After an initial evaluation, the child is entitled to a reevaluation at least every 3 years. The pediatric primary care clinician can suggest that the parent request a reevaluation and can help them review and interpret the relevant findings from this evaluation. This data can provide invaluable information about progress and areas of challenge and help guide decisions regarding special education services. Additionally, this data will provide the pediatric clinician with a detailed overview of the child's developmental and academic strengths and needs. Legal mandates for evaluation are vague, so specific requests from the parent when a child is struggling or not making progress can prompt the school evaluation team to perform a thorough collection of data that inform educational programming.

The Individualized Education Program

The importance of a well-written IEP cannot be overstated, and the pediatric primary care clinician's role in educating the parents about their rights can have a tremendously positive effect on the child's emotional, physical, and developmental outcomes.

Once a child has been found eligible for special education services, an education program is required. The results of the evaluation will be included in the development of the IEP. This document should articulate the strengths of the child; the concerns of the family; the results of the evaluation; the academic, communication, developmental, and functional needs of the child; any behavioral supports necessary; relevance of English proficiency; and if the child is blind or has low vision or is deaf or hard of hearing. For children up to age 3 years, an IFSP is generated with families and will describe a program for home- or child care–based EI, setting measurable goals for the child. Once the child is provided school-based services, an IEP is required.

The IEP must contain the following components:

- **Present level of academic achievement and functional performance (often referred to as the *present level of performance* [PLOP]):** Each IEP should describe in detail the effect of the child's disability on their ability to engage in classroom learning, the social environment, and ADLs. This description should provide a review of the child's present developmental level and ability to perform, areas in which they have progressed, and areas in which they continue to struggle. There should be concrete data that document the level of performance in areas of previously identified concern, and often there is a description of the child's behavior in the classroom.
- **Measurable goals:** The IEP should contain a series of objective and measurable annual and short-term goals that cover a broad base of developmental domains. These targeted areas should include all domains that can be affected by autism: academics, social engagement, language and language pragmatics, play, attentional regulation, flexibility, motor coordination or fine motor skills, and adaptive skills (eg, toileting, dressing, taking care of belongings, transitioning, following instructions). The setting for each area of focus and the specifics of how the goal will be achieved should be a part of the language in the IEP.

  The annual goals of the IEP should address all areas of strength and need identified in the PLOP and define the goals the school plans to address over the academic year. In developing these goals, the team should consider parent concerns and priorities for the child, academic needs or other needs (eg, visual or deaf or hard of hearing needs), testing results if any, and interfering behaviors. The IEP should be developed through a strength-based approach, in which the child's individual strengths are used as a foundation to build on. This type of educational programming has been shown to enhance a child's ability to meet expectations, increase their enthusiasm, and provide opportunities that serve as a benchmark for success.

These goals must be worded in a specific manner to make the goals objective and measurable and to identify the child's present level of functioning. The IEP will define annual goals, but short-term goals should be listed for quarterly progress reports as well. The example of Raul that follows illustrates annual and short-term goals that are objective and measurable. The schools often set goals based on the expectation of how often they are likely to be demonstrated, often using the parameter of the child demonstrating a skill in 3 out of 4 opportunities as a benchmark for completion.

Example: Annual and Short-Term Goals

Raul's present level of performance identifies that he is not yet using words in a functional capacity. He tends to use his body to get his needs met and will push, yell, or grab rather than use words to express himself. An annual goal for Raul may be the following one: "Raul will use words to make requests in lieu of using his body to obtain what he wants." The short-term goals that will help him reach this overall goal should be more specific, objective, and measurable and will build on the success of each goal accomplished.

a. Fall short-term goal: "Raul will use a simple 1- to 2-word verbal phrase such as 'Help,' 'Give me,' or 'My turn' to make requests in structured lessons with a teacher in 3 out of 4 opportunities."
b. Winter short-term goal: "Raul will use simple 1- to 2-word verbal requests throughout the day with a teacher in both structured and unstructured settings in 3 of 4 opportunities."
c. Spring short-term goal: "Raul will use simple 1- to 2-word verbal requests when engaged with peers in free play to ask for a turn or when requesting an object in 3 of 4 opportunities."

This IEP goal dictates that the teacher regularly structure the opportunity to support the child's use of simple verbal requests in lessons and then monitor their progress by collecting data on their success. It states specific short-term goals, beginning with the most proximal and relevant developmental skill. Early learners will make such a request in a specific and structured setting with an adult. As the skill becomes more solid, the child will use these types of requests in different contexts and, later, with a peer and in less structured settings. The goals should evolve to include more mature requests, made across many settings or generalized to different settings that are both structured and unstructured. In the example of Raul, the progression of these parameters reflects a typical developmental continuum for acquiring new skills.

Example: Measurable Goals

The following set of examples illustrates the difference between vague goals and measurable goals:

Vague goal: "Cynthia will improve her reading skills during independent reading time."

Measurable goal: "Given second grade reading materials, Cynthia will read a sentence at 50 words per minute as measured by the Gray Oral Reading Test."

Example: Behavioral Goals

When describing behavioral goals, an understanding of the behavioral triggers, the environmental factors typically involved, and the response of the child's environment or the consequences of the behavior is necessary to set clear and measurable goals in order to ensure progress. The IEP goal designed to teach a child to use verbal requests rather than disruptive behaviors might read as follows:

"On the playground, during unstructured playtime, Juan will use a single word to ask that he 'take a turn' or that a child 'stop' when there is something Juan wants or to object to what another child is doing."

- **Educational progress:** It should be documented how a child's progress is defined and monitored and how often parent(s) will receive progress reports (typically quarterly).
- **Accommodations:** A specific section of the IEP is dedicated to accommodations. It is beneficial for the pediatric primary care clinician to review this section, as accommodations are essential for most children on the autism spectrum. All accommodations necessary for the child's optimal progress should be specified in the appropriate section of the IEP. Most children on the spectrum benefit from accommodations that support communication and executive function skills, at the very least. The following accommodations should be considered for the child and are based on need:
    - Mandated statewide assessments: All children are required to participate in mandated statewide assessments of learning. The IEP specifies which assessments the child will be eligible for and whether the child will receive accommodations, such as individual administration of these assessments. This determination can have long-term effects when placement decisions regarding "diploma track" versus "life skills track" are made in high school.
    - Communication: Use of assistive technology for communication purposes.
    - Books: Use of alternative books, adapted books, extra books for home, or lists of discussion questions.

- Curriculum: Shortened assignments, decreased emphasis on spelling or written work.
- Classroom environment: Removal of distractions, placement of the child proximal to the teacher and boards, use of visual schedules or a computer.
- Directions: Breaking instruction down into individual steps, providing visual reinforcement of instruction, or showing a model of the assignment.
- Time/transitions: Providing additional time for assignments/tests, preparing for transitions, or using a timer.
- Handwriting: Allowing for dictation, offering fill-in response options, allowing briefer responses.
- Testing: Providing a small setting with decreased distractions, having instructions read, allowing more time for assignments.
- Encouragement of on-task behavior: Having the child check in daily with an adult to review what the schedule is and what the child needs for the day, using preferential pairing with a peer who can help by modeling expected behavior, using nonverbal cues with the child, and using positive reinforcement or behavioral incentives with specific goals articulated can all be helpful encouragement.

- **Placement decisions:** Placement decisions cannot be made until the IEP has been written and ratified by the team and the child's parent(s). The parent(s) should understand that they have the right to take documents home, obtain feedback from others, and take their time reviewing these documents before signing an IEP. The IEP does not have to be completed and signed at the meeting. If there is an existing IEP, that IEP will remain active until the new one is completed and signed. Many parents feel overwhelmed by the language in the IEP and the pressure to ratify it. A child's educational placement can be an extremely challenging decision. The law states that the child should be placed into the least restrictive environment, but individual decisions must be made based on services available as well as the child's developmental profile. This part of the process is another opportunity for the pediatric primary care clinician to review relevant areas of the IEP with a family and assist them with decision-making.

  Although access to a general education classroom is ideal for all children, this decision is dependent on the child receiving the support they need to be successful in that environment. If the child is in a general education classroom but is not able to engage with peers or the curriculum, this does not serve the child. Placement decisions should be made carefully, taking into consideration the individual child's past successes and challenges as well as the expertise of the teacher, size of the class, and the child's access to necessary special education services. Additionally, it is important that the parent(s) understand what type of special educator will be available and how many children they will be serving in addition to their child. The IEP will state the total number of hours during which the child will receive special education support, but some services may be administered by an instructional aide rather than a special educator. This aide could be responsible for many other children with IEPs as well. A placement determination should be made after careful review and never based solely on a diagnosis or a family's preference.

Once an overall placement decision is made, decisions about all individual classes and the number of hours of services are made. A child placed into a general education setting could be pulled out of that setting for special education services, or a child placed into an autism self-contained classroom might spend time in a general education classroom for social engagement or for classes in which they are able to have access to the grade-level curriculum. A chart in the IEP lists both the placement and the number of special education hours. The pediatric primary care clinician can assist the parent(s) in understanding this process and be certain they are in full agreement that these placement and service determinations are in the best interest of their child.

- **Extended school year (ESY) services:** Each year, the IEP team will determine whether the child is eligible for schooling during the school break. Summer programming does not necessarily take place in the same school or with familiar staff. It is of variable length and is typically reserved for the children not making expected progress. The school evaluation team may not recommend ESY services if a child might be placed with children who have more severe educational delays. Recommendations vary from one school system to another.
- **Independent educational evaluations (IEEs):** A parent has the right to an IEE at public expense if there is significant disagreement about the results or interpretation of an evaluation made by the school. This can be especially important when the family does not have the financial resources to seek private services and there is disagreement about a diagnosis, eligibility, or recommendations for services being made. In addition, an IEE may be indicated if a more detailed assessment is required by a specialist or private psychologist to resolve the dispute. The parent is then empowered to find a specialist in the private community or from the approved list who might have more specific expertise in psychological assessment or behavioral intervention and can therefore serve as a consultant to the team. The contexts in which an IEE might be of benefit include behavioral challenges that are not responding to intervention, lack of developmental progress, or a dispute over services, diagnosis, or placement.

The IEP document should be used to review and monitor a child's developmental and educational progress, set the stage for educational goals and services, and determine which accommodations should be put into place. The IEP is a legal document with which the school is required by law to comply. Noncompliance, or the lack of progress in the areas described in an IEP, requires a higher level of intervention or services. A clearly stated IEP can provide assurance should the parents become concerned about their child's progress in school. The pediatric primary care clinician can encourage the parents to request modifications to the IEP when appropriate. If the child is not meeting their IEP goals, the school may be required to provide more services or change the child's placement (potentially requiring a private school placement at public expense). Without a clearly written IEP, the child and family have little recourse if the child struggles.

The pediatric primary care clinician should aim to review a child's IEP annually with the family to assess the adequacy of the breadth and depth of services. In situations where there is a significant discrepancy between the primary care clinician's and parents' ideas and those of the school, the family may benefit from working with a private educational advocate to assist with the process of IEP writing, participation in IEP meetings, and review of eligible services. The Council of Parent Attorneys and Advocates offers lists of licensed advocates by region (www.copaa.org/page/Direct). Family Voices may be an additional resource for families (https://familyvoices.org). Alternatively, one of the child's private therapists could serve as the child's advocate with the school. Lawyers are rarely needed unless a child's case has moved to mediation over disputes. Additionally, there are local nonprofit organizations that offer advocacy assistance and education about parental rights, such as the Center for Parent Information and Resources (www.parentcenterhub.org/find-your-center).

The pediatric primary care clinician should become familiar with the formatting used in IEPs within their school districts. Each IEP document has a section where important demographic and process information is found. The educational diagnosis the school is using to find the child eligible for services is found in this section. In the early preschool years, the IEP team may use a vague eligibility, such as "developmental delay," but as the child ages, a specific diagnosis that meets the state's eligibility requirements for services is needed. It is preferable that the school use an autism eligibility as soon as possible to ensure broad-based services and avoid limitation of services to only one or a few particular areas of concern.

The IEP's demographic sheet specifies when the last full psychoeducational evaluation was completed and when the next one is due (in a maximum of 3 years). In some cases, the IEP team may decide that a reevaluation is unnecessary when the child continues to require special education services or is determined to no longer need these services. The pediatric primary care clinician should remind parents that it remains their legal right to insist on this reevaluation regardless of whether the team feels it may be useful. Documenting a child's psychological and academic progress is imperative. Data points are more predictive when followed over time rather than when measured at a single point in time. These psychological data help define a child's progress and areas of need and will be used to guide revision of educational programming. Without the documentation of performance, parents have no right to request services. Parents should be encouraged to track the data over time.

The pediatric primary care clinician would do well to remind parents that this reevaluation should consist of a full set of data collected every 3 years, including psychological or cognitive data, educational performance, and specific areas of concern: language and communication, self-regulation, ADLs, motor skills, and whatever else is relevant to the child's needs.

The box at the end of this chapter lists resources available to parents to educate themselves and receive support in the IEP process. Many families benefit from working with a private educational advocate or a local nonprofit advocacy group to help define areas to target in the IEP, discuss strategies for reaching these goals, assist with writing the IEP, and attend meetings with the family. Parents should be advised to always bring one other person to all IEP meetings to take notes and support the family.

The Annual Individualized Education Program Review

The pediatric primary care clinician should aim to review a child's IEP with the parents on an annual basis. There are ample opportunities for the primary care clinician to support the parents as they continue to advocate for their child's needs. Parents should be instructed to share a copy of their child's most recently completed IEP with their child's primary care clinician, who can save the document in the electronic health record. This IEP can serve as the basis for review of a child's progress over the year, and parents should be made aware that sharing it is a priority for case management within the medical home. A great deal of information about the child can be extracted from the IEP. The pediatric primary care clinician can play an important role in helping guide the process as services and goals are determined and placement decisions are made each year. The IEP meeting can be an overwhelming time for a family, so reviewing a draft or the prior year's IEP with a professional (the pediatric primary care clinician or a therapist involved in the child's care) can help parents prepare and organize their thoughts for upcoming meetings. Families should be aware that involvement in this special education process is a priority for pediatric clinicians.

Educating parents about the ways in which they can further advocate for their child in the special education process can be extremely useful. Parents should know that the IEP can be modified at any point without a full IEP meeting if there are concerns about the child's progress or if the child has met their goals before the end of the IEP's 12-month period.

Although it would be unusual for a primary care clinician to attend an IEP meeting, if the clinician is motivated to do so, they can provide tremendous support to the family. Attendance can often be remote, and there are *Current Procedural Terminology* codes (under "team conference" codes **99366**, **99367**, or **99368**) available to charge for medical team conference with an interdisciplinary team. (Reimbursement is variable.) Involvement in this process provides a valuable advocacy opportunity and provides tremendous support for patients and their families.

CASE VIGNETTE: CONCLUSION

Evan's parents schedule an appointment to consult with his primary care clinician about the school's recommendations for his second grade year. His parents express concern that the IEP team has proposed withdrawing special education support. They observe that Evan still struggles in many ways and is not able to integrate successfully without support. They share that he has many restricted and repetitive behaviors and interests and that he struggles with conversational exchange and peer play. He shows inflexibility when interacting, and many peers lose interest in him. Evan's parents additionally note that when they read him books, he is interested in certain ideas and pictures but is not always attentive to the main theme of the book. He will struggle to retell a story or answer questions about the ideas in the book. Further, they have noted he is struggling with math word problems and the language-based learning involved in science class. They seek the primary care clinician's advice on how best to proceed.

Evan's primary care clinician begins by raising the importance of a new psychoeducational evaluation, which is Evan's right as described in his IEP. The clinician instructs the parents that Evan's prior IEP remains valid until they sign a new one and shares that they should not feel pressure to do so until they feel satisfied with Evan's educational plan. Further, the primary care clinician advises Evan's parents not to sign the new recommendations and asks the family if they are able to consult with a private advocate, an advocacy group, or a therapist who has worked with Evan and could attend the IEP meeting with them. The school subsequently agrees to perform a new evaluation at the request of Evan's parents.

The primary care clinician then provides Evan's parents with a list of the developmental areas they should request be included in the evaluation: a measure of verbal and nonverbal intelligence, educational testing, a full language evaluation, evaluation of adaptive behaviors, a behavioral observation, and autism-specific screening completed by all teachers and parents. The pediatric primary care clinician recommends a private psychological evaluation, should the IEP team not agree to an evaluation. The family puts Evan on a wait list for this evaluation in anticipation of needing guidance from a more comprehensive evaluation.

The assessment data collected by the school are reviewed at an IEP meeting, and the team discusses that Evan has many cognitive and educational strengths. Evan performs in the average range for nonverbal IQ and in many academic areas, except for reading comprehension. His language pragmatics and his verbal IQ are in the low range. He has strengths in information, vocabulary, and digit span (repeating sequences of numbers), but his verbal comprehension and similarities are in the low range. His autism questionnaire supports the diagnosis of autism and persistent behavioral concerns that are affecting his classroom participation. Analysis of questionnaire results demonstrate difficulties in social-emotional reciprocity, peer socialization, restricted behavior, atypical language, and attention. A review of ADLs reveals that he requires prompting to use the toilet and to follow everyday routines.

The IEP team meets again for eligibility and finds that Evan qualifies for continued educational support while he is placed within a general education setting, with the following IEP goals and supports:

- Social skills class for social reciprocity and language pragmatics
- Classroom goals of story retelling, language pragmatics and comprehension, peer socialization, and transitions
- Special education support in the general education classroom for academic lessons (15 hours per week)
- Positive behavior plan focusing on attention to tasks and nonpreferred activities
- Use of visual aids to support adaptive behaviors, including toileting and independence with daily routines

The clinician should strive to ensure that each child has an IEP that includes educating the child in the least restrictive environment with optimal professional services specific to the child's unique challenges. There are many opportunities for the pediatric primary care clinician to help support parents as they advocate for their child's needs. Educational goals should be broad based and include all developmental domains relevant to autism and the child. The goal is to address as many barriers as possible to the child's optimal developmental course and to enable the child to become an independent adult engaged in their community.

Clinical Pearls

- There are many opportunities for the pediatric primary care clinician to have a role in educating families and advocating for a child's rights within the special education system.
- The pediatric primary care clinician should review the IEP with the family annually.
- The pediatric primary care clinician has a role in the following parts of the process:
  - Recommend initial screening and evaluation for children in whom developmental delays and/or atypical developmental processes are a concern.
  - Educate parents about which types of professionals and evaluations should be requested on the initial and 3-year evaluations.
  - Help ensure that the IEP adequately describes the child's current level of performance while identifying relevant strengths and needs.
  - Ensure that the IEP has a broad set of goals with both annual and short-term objectives that are measurable.

Continued on next page

— Consider whether the use of an educational advocate is indicated or possible to support the IEP process.
— Ensure there is a detailed description in the IEP of the child's required accommodations.
— Review progress reports with the family to ensure that data on the child's progress are being collected in the classroom.

Parent Resources: The Individualized Education Program Process

- Twachtman-Cullen D, Twachtman-Reilly J. *How Well Does Your IEP Measure Up? Quality Indicators for Effective Service Delivery.* Starfish Specialty Press; 2003
- US Department of Education. Office of Special Education Programs (OSEP). Accessed March 3, 2026. https://www2.ed.gov/about/offices/list/osers/osep/index.html?src=mr
- Weinfeld R, Davis M. *Special Needs Advocacy Resource Book: What You Can Do Now to Advocate for Your Exceptional Child's Education.* Prufrock Press; 2008
- Wright PW, Wright PD. Wrightslaw. Accessed March 3, 2026. https://www.wrightslaw.com (free online resource for special education processes)
- Wright PW, Wright PD. *Wrightslaw: Special Education Law.* 3rd ed. Harbor House Law Press; 2023

References

Cartwright JD; American Academy of Pediatrics Council on Children With Disabilities. Provision of educationally related services for children and adolescents with chronic diseases and disabling conditions. *Pediatrics.* 2007;119(6):1218–1223 PMID: 17545394 doi: 10.1542/peds.2007-0885

Gereige TS, Zenni EA, eds. *School Health: Policy and Practice.* 7th ed. American Academy of Pediatrics; 2016 doi: 10.1542/9781581108453

CHAPTER 15

Long-Term Goals and Transition Planning: It Takes a Village

CASE VIGNETTE

Alexander was 2 years old when he received an autism diagnosis. His family developed a relationship with a pediatric clinician who was interested in family-focused care for children with developmental disabilities. The clinician spoke with the family at regular visits about Alexander's developmental progress and the goals his parents had identified. They regularly reviewed his individualized education program (IEP), indicators for outside private therapies, and the family's pursuit of activities in their community that built on his strengths.

Alexander received services in a self-contained autism preschool setting and worked privately with an applied behavior analysis therapist during the preschool years. The work tended to focus on teaching flexibility, transitioning, attending to nonpreferred activities, and engaging in peer play and interaction. Alexander's developmental skills were progressing nicely, although he used very few words to communicate. He was able to transition successfully into kindergarten while initially being placed into a special education classroom.

Alexander had minimal verbal communication and, over his first year, began to exhibit some externalizing and disruptive behaviors (to his functioning and others' space). An assessment for augmentative and alternative communication (AAC) and a functional behavioral assessment were performed and it was clear that Alexander would benefit from using an augmentative form of communication rather than relying on oral communication. The IEP team found he was able to use an electronic device with a communication app that was adapted for his use, so his parents were eager to learn and incorporate this device at home. Alexander could initially communicate with only single words

Continued on next page

using the AAC device, but as he developed expertise, the app allowed him to combine frequently used words and advance to using complete sentences with the speech-generating component. Alexander became more regulated and adaptable as he was successful in using the AAC device to communicate.

Over the subsequent years, Alexander spent time in general education classes with ample accommodations and special education support. His educational programming allowed for direct teaching of independence skills in addition to his academics. Alexander's parents capitalized on his interests in the natural world and animals, and he joined a Boy Scouts troop where he was welcomed by his peers as the expert on plant identification. In high school, Alexander was placed into a life skills program where he was encouraged to pursue his interests in addition to the academic curricula. He attended a social skills class that focused on engaging in conversational exchange and expressing and learning strategies for managing emotions. He also learned about safety, dating and sexuality, and self-advocacy.

After high school, Alexander's parents identified a veterinarian who invited him to have a supervised internship at the office. Alexander was given jobs that accessed his cognitive skills: arranging supplies, identifying expired medications, taking animals on walks, and assisting in other ways in the office. When he graduated from high school, the veterinarian hired him as an office assistant. He had a list of daily job expectations and checked in with an office administrator at the beginning and end of each day. He knew he could approach this person if he was having difficulty and learned to find a quiet place where he could go to calm and self-regulate if needed. His parents continued to enroll him in social skills programming to supply him with additional life skills. The family and Alexander hope he will one day be able to live in a supervised apartment with other young adults. The family attended sessions at a local nonprofit organization about financial planning and special needs trusts for children and adults with disabilities. Alexander has discovered People First for Young Adults, a national resource providing transition services for young adults, where he is part of a peer group, learns more life skills, and is building relationships and getting support from other young adults with disabilities.

This book has focused on ways pediatric primary care clinicians can play a pivotal role in improving outcomes for children on the autism spectrum and their families. It has explored the definition and presentation of autism, emphasizing the importance of early identification and diagnosis. Later chapters highlighted ways primary care clinicians can advocate for early, comprehensive, evidence-based interventions and environmental accommodations while addressing co-occurring conditions that may hinder a child's development and well-being.

Autism is not something to be cured, nor is there an expectation that individuals on the spectrum become indistinguishable from their peers. People on the spectrum are not broken; they do not need fixing. The neurodiversity perspective recognizes that human brains function in diverse ways and that autistic individuals simply experience and interact with the world differently than neurotypical individuals. The goal of primary care management is to learn from the social model, which emphasizes partnering with families to create supportive environments that foster community participation and inclusion for their children.

Parents will at some point ask about long-term expectations for their child on the spectrum. Many parents hope their child will outgrow the autism diagnosis, they will "catch up" developmentally to their typically developing peers, or they will be able to mask or hide their atypical features so they can blend in with the neurotypical world. Other families embrace and accept their child and have an ease about finding ways to celebrate their strengths. They appreciate that their child may progress developmentally at a pace or on a path that is not the one expected of a neurotypical child. This chapter addresses how the pediatric primary care clinician can be involved in the child's evolution while supporting the family in developing objectives and realistic expectations that support the long-term life goals for individuals on the spectrum. It is the primary care clinician who has the opportunity to provide the support, empathy, and optimism that will benefit families as they navigate their child's life.

The Data on Outcomes

Longitudinal research data demonstrate that most individuals who receive an autism diagnosis will continue to meet criteria for this diagnosis throughout their lifespan. It is important to mention that these data are limited by the populations they have studied. There are likely many individuals with a broader phenotype who were not included in either diagnosis or longitudinal analysis and who are therefore not represented in these research findings. The populations represented by the literature are those that have access to specialists and can be evaluated for diagnosis and may represent those with more significant developmental challenges or co-occurring conditions. There may be others that are able to progress academically, socially, and independently later in life without special education support or individualized therapy. These individuals may still experience challenges in social functioning or communication or co-occurring behavioral health conditions. Their outcomes may differ from those who received a diagnosis earlier, yet this group is likely to be underrepresented in research literature.

Meta-analyses continue to show that approximately 20% of autistic adults will require only minimal support with a high level of independence in work, home, and social engagement; 31%, regular support with engagement through scheduled activities; and 48%, daily support in a specialized residential facility. The majority of adults who have received an autism diagnosis (61% in Australia and 87% in the United States) continue to live with their families. Only 33% of all adults on the autism spectrum will be employed. Those with an average to above-average intelligence quotient (IQ) as well as strengths in adaptive skills are more likely to obtain and maintain employment. Adults on the spectrum, more than individuals with other disabilities and cognitive challenges, continue to experience difficulties with social reciprocity and relational intimacy and are more likely to withdraw from socializing with others. In studies where community engagement is supported, individuals on the spectrum tend to have fewer intimate relationships than other adults with disabilities.

These research data are sobering, but individual studies using newer methods of job training, supervision, mentoring, and use of technologies and supports for autistic adults in the workplace offer more promise. Additional opportunities with employers that have prioritized hiring adults with disabilities have created opportunities and adapted expectations that are more inclusive of individuals on the spectrum and allow for more success in the workplace. These methods are reviewed in the list of transition planning components in the next section of this chapter, Long-Term and Transition Planning. Individuals with the earlier establishment of an autism diagnosis and earlier entrance into therapeutic settings using evidence-based treatments and parental involvement show improved success in achieving partial independence, better communication skills, higher educational levels, and the ability to live independently. Other early predictors of independence in adults are an average to above-average IQ, strengths in verbal skills in the preschool years, and strengths in motor imitation. Of particular interest and relevance to long-term planning, it was found that children on the spectrum who had the opportunity for community engagement and inclusion in the school setting during their childhood were more likely to have more success with relational intimacy, employment, community engagement, and independence as adults. This finding supports the involvement of the primary care clinician in promoting inclusion as a lifetime goal in the child's care.

Further, it is important to restate that autism is a type of neurodivergence that by definition is extremely heterogeneous in its phenotype. More recent research identifies that when employers have an awareness of the needs of the individual with a disability or neurodivergence and can create more inclusive and supportive work environments that are supportive of these differences, the individual is more likely to experience long-term success in the workplace. Autistic individuals are likely to require support around communication challenges, feelings of isolation, and lack of engagement with peers and supervisors. This type of support will be helpful in teaching individuals to process experiences of frustrations, stress, and perceived failure in the workplace. Creating jobs that rely on the strengths of the autistic individual and making accommodations to avoid exacerbations of underlying sensory issues, communication challenges, or anxiety offer promise for increasing levels of productivity and retention for those with neurodivergence. Ensuring employment will further support the individual's sense of belonging and self-efficacy, and efforts to enable this should be a part of long-term planning for the child.

Long-Term and Transition Planning

The process of setting individualized long-term goals for each child on the autism spectrum begins at diagnosis and continues throughout the child's life. The pediatric primary care clinician plays a key role in this process, starting this process by aiding the family to understand the meaning of an autism diagnosis and find appropriate therapies. The idea of a lifelong process of planning for the child's growth will be revisited during each subsequent appointment. It is essential that the family not only understand and accept the diagnosis but also find supports and therapies that are appropriate for their child and address a wide range of developmental goals over the long term. The use of a strength-based approach with each child, discussed in Chapter 1, Caring for the Autistic Child in the Medical Home, serves as an effective way to motivate both child and family, foster trust and optimism, and collaboratively establish meaningful goals for the child's educational and therapeutic planning. It is important to understand that each child will have a different trajectory of development, so planning will need to be adjusted to meet the individual needs of the child and their family.

The clinician will optimally engage in conversations with the family at various stages of the child's life to assess progress, adjust treatment goals, and create needed accommodations to the environment. Transition planning for adulthood is a long-term endeavor aimed at helping the individual reach the highest possible level of independence and community involvement. The plan must therefore identify the necessary supports and treatment objectives to foster the child's independence, well-being, and productivity.

Following are the components of successful long-term planning and transition planning:

- **Ongoing evaluation and adaptation of the systems that serve youth on the spectrum:** This process requires careful attention to the policies, practices, and procedures that promote equity in service access and support for these youth. The professionals caring for the autistic child must receive adequate training and develop an awareness of the potential bias existing toward those on the spectrum. They will need to ensure there is a successful method for communication with the child and family so a collaborative process for decision-making and the development of accommodations are achieved over the lifespan.
- **Early establishment of an autism diagnosis:** Chapters 5, Autism Screening in Primary Care, and 6, Establishing the Autism Diagnosis, discuss screening for and diagnosis of autism. The approach is to identify behaviors that suggest autism, make early diagnoses, and subsequently refer for appropriate therapy. No longer should a "wait and watch" approach be accepted, as early intervention has resulted in better outcomes for young children on the spectrum.

- **Early and intensive intervention with an emphasis on communication:** Regardless of the developmental challenges identified, it is important that there be a focus on teaching the use of language (either spoken language or forms of AAC; refer to Chapter 8, Evidence-Based Supports and Services, for more information) for communication purposes. Teaching the pragmatics of getting needs met, initiating conversation, staying on the topic of conversation, and learning to sustain exchanges of communication on a maintained topic will ensure success with social engagement and learning.
- **Teaching skills of independence across all settings (school, home, and community) beginning at diagnosis:** Mastering activities of daily living helps children build a sense of competence and fosters their independence both at home and in the community. These skills of daily living, or *adaptive behaviors,* are directly linked to the autistic adult's ability to live independently. They begin with elementary skills around toileting, hygiene, and transitioning and later evolve to skills required of adults to live independently (eg, financial literacy, sexuality and dating, use of various modes of transportation, cooking, reading schedules). Autism treatment programs, public school life skills programs, and community assistance programs place a priority on teaching skills of functional independence and are staffed by professionals with expertise in this area. It is important that the individuals on the spectrum who do not require the more intensive level of special education support also have access to this type of programming to ready them for adult independence. Standardized assessments to identify need can be performed at each developmental level and should be included in IEPs.
- **Educating the child's peers about the child's specific needs:** It can be particularly effective to suggest to parents that they or the teacher prepare their child's peers so they understand the autistic child's behaviors and learn ways they can be supportive. In general, typically developing children and adults will be more available to support an individual if they have this understanding or are invited to model desired behaviors for the child. An example of how a request can be made to a classmate to teach, through modeling, the child with a disability or neurodivergence may be "This is Arjun. He does not always use words to share when he needs something. If you could be a good friend by asking if he needs help when he seems to have difficulty or modeling for him how to use words, he will be more likely to learn how to do it."
- **Including the child's interests in choices and decision-making:** The pediatric primary care clinician can be instrumental in advising parents to make choices for their child based on their strengths and likely success in a particular activity. The child is more likely to be included by their peers and be motivated to work hard if they feel competent. This competency will foster the child's perception of self-worth.

- **Teaching functional social and communication skills, how to build and maintain friendships, how to date, and self-awareness around emotional regulation and problem-solving:** Finding opportunities for successful engagement with peers as early as possible can lead to the building of social connections that result in more independence in adulthood. In the preschool years, this is likely to be a part of the treatment plan for the child, but as a case manager, the primary care clinician should ensure that this goal continues to be prioritized throughout the lifespan. There are curricula for teaching social skills in the school and in private therapies, and the clinician should work with families to use the child's strengths to create opportunities for engagement with others. The primary care clinician can assess a child's IEP and private therapies to look for an opportunity for teaching social engagement. Educators and social skills specialists are familiar with teaching strategies to support the development of social skills. For example, a simple curriculum is described in Kasari's Remaking Recess research. This program provides a structure for play to support interaction. The teacher prepares the children by providing a specific activity with assigned roles, rules, and props. This has been shown to result in more peer-to-peer interactions. Kasari's program proposes the use of playground equipment for two and the use of peer modeling to teach social interaction in order to set the stage for progressive levels of inclusion. Some programs for social engagement teach perspective taking to alert a child to understand how their behavior affects others. Other programs include teaching concrete skills for successful conversational exchange, teaching lessons about sexuality, providing dating and intimacy advice, and exploring other pragmatic social skills. The primary care clinician can encourage the parent to inquire about availability for this type of programming in their school and community.
- **Identifying recreational and social activities:** The pediatric primary care clinician should create and maintain lists of adaptive and inclusive recreational and other activities within their community. Autism Speaks and local autism parent groups can offer support with resources. There are likely to be a variety of resources available (eg, scouting, martial arts, drama, music, and arts) through community and parent-run groups, private schools, private providers, and therapists that focus on both adaptive forms of recreation and opportunities in which autistic children can be included with typical peers. The primary care clinician can encourage parents to find resources to assist with identifying these types of peer engagement.
- **Finding peer groups:** Most communities will provide opportunity for peer groups. As with all children, forming relationships with peers who have similar developmental profiles, strengths, and interests will boost an autistic child's sense of connection and self-worth.

- **Addressing safety issues including elopement, self-injurious behavior, aggression, drowning, injuries, substance use, and bullying:** Individuals on the spectrum are at increased risk for fatal injuries such as drowning, falls, and motor vehicle–pedestrian collisions. Thoughtful planning is required to teach the young child to swim and to practice street and stranger safety, while putting protective safety measures into place in all settings. Childproof locks, secure screens, alarms on doors, and gates in the backyard are essential for some children. Many community police departments have specific programs that train officers to approach an autistic individual who is in distress without causing escalation. Having these individuals wear GPS tracking devices, an ID band, or an autism safety card can be lifesaving. Suggestions such as these are available as resources through national and local autism parent groups, several of which are listed in **Box 15.1**. Registering an autistic child with the police department and including constructive guidance on how to approach the child are also helpful. This approach ensures that officers and department staff are aware of the child's profile and location.

  Children who have difficulties with reading social cues and communication are at significant risk of being bullied. Children on the spectrum who are placed into general education environments may have minimal special education

BOX 15.1 Autism Advocacy Supports for Families

- Association for Autism and Neurodiversity (https://aane.org): A service organization that provides education and support for autistic and neurodivergent people and their families as well as for professionals involved in care.
- Autism Society (https://autismsociety.org): An organization committed to advocacy and creating community and providing resources for autistic individuals and their families.
- The ARC (https://thearc.org): The national hub for searching for local chapters dedicated to advocacy, financial planning, special education support, and employment training and long-term support for people with intellectual and developmental disabilities.
- Center for Parent Information and Resources (www.parentcenterhub.org/find-your-center): The national hub for regional centers for parent information and resources for children with developmental differences.
- MyAutismTeam (www.myautismteam.com): A social network platform offering autistic individuals and their families an opportunity to connect and share information.
- Organization for Autism Research (https://researchautism.org): An organization that supports research on the challenges faced by autistic individuals and their families and provides supports across the lifespan, including peer groups, education, and job placement support.
- Parent-run nonprofit organizations: Each state has its own such organization offering autism support for families. Examples include DC Autism Parents (www.dcautismparents.org), POAC Autism Services in New Jersey (www.poac.net) and Parents of Autistic Children of Northern Virginia (https://poac-nova.org).

support, so bullying may go unnoticed. The pediatric primary care clinician should ask about bullying regularly and advise parents about the need for heightened awareness and intervention when there is concern so that any incidences of bullying can be addressed early.

- **Identifying and treating medical, psychiatric, and behavioral health coexisting conditions:** Earlier chapters (Chapters 10, Diagnosing and Managing Co-Occurring Conditions; 11, Gastrointestinal Symptoms and Feeding Challenges; and 12, Insomnia: Identification and Interventions) focus on the importance of the early identification and treatment of coexisting conditions in autism. Substance use disorders and concomitant psychiatric illness (anxiety, depression, mood instability, and schizophrenia) add to the long-term complexity of outcomes for individuals on the spectrum. The pediatric primary care clinician can be pivotal in supporting proactive interventions to promote healthy lifestyles and recognizing the need and referring for treatment as they would for any child.
- **Continuing with a strength-based approach to find opportunities for community engagement:** Using a strength-based approach to working with a child on the spectrum not only motivates the child more but calls on strengths to create opportunity for learning and engagement. A child interested in order and arranging might find an opportunity to organize materials. One such vocational training opportunity put selected young adults on the spectrum into medical settings where they could arrange the medications in order of expiration date. A child with technical proficiency might find an opportunity with the theater technical department. Another child with precocious number skills might lead bingo games with elderly people or keep statistics for the sports team. The child who has an interest in plants and animals might find an opportunity to work on a farm or for a veterinarian or to engage with scouting. An individual with an interest in dinosaurs might volunteer at the museum of natural history. Those with musical talent may participate in community orchestras or theaters. Individuals with math skills might excel in chess, robotics, or engineering clubs.
- **Providing necessary supports and preparing for each life transition:** All children struggle during necessary transitions, and the pediatric primary care clinician can be helpful in discussing how best to support this process. The autistic child will be especially vulnerable when expectations change, the routines and environment change, and the new educational team does not know the child. It will be important to provide a transition plan and prepare for what may be expected after the transition. If the child is at a pivotal point developmentally and there is a plan to decrease support, clinicians should advise the family to allow for the transition first, before making significant changes in special education support, and to have the plan written in the IEP and approved by the family.

- **Including the individual on the spectrum in decision-making:** Including the child in important discussions such as IEP meetings, the creation of behavior plans, and transition planning supports the processes of self-determination and self-advocacy. The autistic child benefits from being given opportunities to learn about their own individual strengths and challenges. Including the child in educational planning and decision-making as early as possible is recommended to develop these skills. Further, in the office, the primary care clinician should include the child, when relevant, in the discussion about their progress and need for support. In these ways, the child can develop valuable skills of self-awareness and self-advocacy.
- **Teaching self-awareness and problem-solving to support self-advocacy:** At some point, autistic children will begin to notice that they are treated differently than their peers. Parents should be guided by their child's pediatric primary care clinician, therapists, and educators to teach their child about their autism diagnosis. If the child has adequate verbal skills, parents can point out to the child their strengths while being realistic about their need for support. Teaching the child about the variable expressions of brain development and how these expressions are manifested in each individual's strengths and challenges can be helpful. Providing the parents with language to teach a child about the variety of human behaviors and how autism fits into that spectrum of expressions can be a helpful model. Ultimately, it is important that the child be educated about their strengths and areas of challenge so they can be effective self-advocates. There are many resources, peer support groups, parent support groups, and nonprofit groups that can serve to guide families in having constructive discussions with children about their autism (refer to the "Transition Planning Resources for Families" box at the end of this chapter).

  All children benefit from learning self-advocacy skills. The autistic child may not understand and express their own needs. They may struggle with problem-solving and flexibility, so it is imperative these types of skills be a part of the treatment plan throughout the lifespan. The primary care clinician can discuss the need for teaching these types of life skills to the parents and child at regular intervals. Priority may be placed on teaching a child to learn how to ask for help, articulate what they are experiencing, express when they are stressed, and how to regulate their emotions. These skills lead to resilience and more effective problem-solving that will serve them well when facing challenges.
- **Obtaining publicly funded financial assistance:** There are many publicly funded assistance options, including Medicaid waivers and the Social Security Administration Supplemental Security Income. In addition, the family should establish a special needs trust for the child to allow the individual to receive income while still meeting criteria for publicly funded financing. Medicaid waivers are distributed through each state based on medical need and not family finances. Families should be advised by the pediatric primary care

clinician or another professional involved in their child's care to work with nonprofit organizations such as The Arc (https://thearc.org), social services, or a special needs attorney to learn about the financial resources that will be helpful for adult life.

- **Preparing for employment opportunities and teaching the skills required:** Individuals on the spectrum may require additional supports to prepare for and maintain employment, such as visual schedules; a clear description of the job and details of its responsibilities, routines, and expected behavior; on-site training; ongoing mentoring; positive behavior supports; and a thorough description of supportive accommodations. Many adults on the spectrum have the cognitive ability to be successful but may not have the ease and fluidity of social pragmatics and communication that make interactions in the workplace easy. They may experience others making assumptions about their abilities and perhaps being exclusive and/or judgmental. Finding employers that have created opportunities for individuals with neurodivergence and are aware of what types of environmental modifications can support the individual is ideal. A search for supportive workplaces through word-of-mouth referrals from other neurodivergent individuals or from professionals with relevant experience can be helpful. Some families may develop relationships with people at potential work environments who can be educated to provide the supports necessary. Many of the advocacy resources listed in **Box 15.1** can link families and individuals to workplace support and trainings. These workplaces will optimally have an understanding of the potential areas of vulnerability an individual on the spectrum may have (eg, sensory processing difficulties, communication challenges, anxiety, difficulties with social interaction). The aim is to match a job opportunity to the cognitive strengths of the individual and determine which types of accommodations will help them be comfortable and effective in the job for which they are hired. A plethora of technologies and apps provide support with executive function skills, self-regulation, and communication skills in adults on the spectrum and can serve to reduce the amount of support required. These supports may be offered as part of job preparedness programming available through the public schools or university-based programs.

Conclusion

This final chapter has explored many different areas in which the pediatric primary care clinician can intervene during a child's lifetime to help prepare them for life's transitions, both daily and major ones. The case vignette at the start of this chapter provides ample examples of how the primary care clinician can provide this type of support throughout the child's lifespan. The process begins at diagnosis, when a family and child first begin to learn what autism is, and then continues as the areas for growth are delineated and discussed at each visit. Including the child in this process is very effective when teaching the child self-awareness and advocacy.

There will be many opportunities for the clinician to intervene and discuss ways to plan proactively in anticipation of life transitions and challenges to optimize long-term outcomes for the adult.

This guide has introduced a variety of ways in which the pediatric primary care clinician can be integrally involved in case management for the autistic child. Many clinical checklists, tools, and resources are provided to assist with this process to make it more accessible to the general clinician. The clinician will not only find new opportunities for learning about autism but also discover ways to become intimately involved with families as they support their children on the journey of autism. The primary care clinician is encouraged to become incrementally more involved in reviewing the autistic child's progress and guiding families as they make decisions about their child's care over the lifespan.

This guide was written to be used as a resource with both a review of the research literature and a collection of practical suggestions and tools that will allow the pediatric primary care clinician to integrate the care of the autistic child into everyday pediatric care. The hope is that although there is much to learn, there is a significant opportunity to positively affect care and outcomes for children on the autism spectrum and their families and a personal sense of reward for this work, both of which will make this effort worthwhile.

Transition Planning Resources for Families

- The Arc of Northern Virginia. *Securing a Future for Your Child With a Disability: A Guide to Transitioning From High School to Adult Services for Adults With Disabilities in Alexandria, Arlington, Fairfax & Falls Church.* 2019. Accessed March 3, 2026. https://thearcofnova.org/wp-content/uploads/sites/6/2018/11/Securing-a-Future-October-2019.pdf
- Larson EM. *I Am Utterly Unique: Celebrating the Strengths of Children with Asperger Syndrome and High-Functioning Autism.* Autism Asperger Publishing Co; 2006
- Transition to adulthood. Autism Speaks. Accessed March 3, 2026. https://www.autismspeaks.org/information-topic#transition
- Verdick E, Reeve E. *The Survival Guide for Kids with Autism Spectrum Disorders (and Their Parents).* Free Spirit Publishing; 2012

References

Donvan J, Zucker C. Autism's first child. *Atlantic.* October 2010. Accessed March 3, 2026. https://www.theatlantic.com/magazine/archive/2010/10/autisms-first-child/308227

Harstad E, Hanson E, Brewster SJ, et al. Persistence of autism spectrum disorder from early childhood through school age. *JAMA Pediatr.* 2023;177(11):1197–1205 PMID: 37782510 doi: 10.1001/jamapediatrics.2023.4003

Kretzmann M, Shih W, Kasari C. Improving peer engagement of children with autism on the school playground: a randomized controlled trial. *Behav Ther.* 2015;46(1):20–28 PMID: 25526832 doi: 10.1016/j.beth.2014.03.006

Magiati I, Tay XW, Howlin P. Cognitive, language, social and behavioural outcomes in adults with autism spectrum disorders: a systematic review of longitudinal follow-up studies in adulthood. *Clin Psychol Rev.* 2014;34(1):73–86 PMID: 24424351 doi: 10.1016/j.cpr.2013.11.002

Nicholas DB, Klag M. Critical reflections on employment among autistic adults. *Autism Adulthood.* 2020;2(4):289–295 PMID: 36600962 doi: 10.1089/aut.2020.0006

Poon KK, Sidhu DJ. Adults with autism spectrum disorders: a review of outcomes, social attainment, and interventions. *Curr Opin Psychiatry.* 2017;30(2):77–84 PMID: 28009723 doi: 10.1097/YCO.0000000000000306

Posar A, Visconti P. Long-term outcome of autism spectrum disorder. *Turk Pediatri Ars.* 2019;54(4):207–212 PMID: 31949411 doi: 10.14744/TurkPediatriArs.2019.16768

Weitzman C, Nadler C, Blum NJ, Augustyn M; Supporting Access for Everyone Consensus Panel. Health care for youth with neurodevelopmental disabilities: a consensus statement. *Pediatrics.* 2024;153(5):e2023063809 PMID: 38596852 doi: 10.1542/peds.2023-063809

White PH, Cooley WC; Transitions Clinical Report Authoring Group; American Academy of Pediatrics, American Academy of Family Physicians, American College of Physicians. Supporting the health care transition from adolescence to adulthood in the medical home. *Pediatrics.* 2018;142(5):e20182587 PMID: 30348754 doi: 10.1542/peds.2018-2587

APPENDIX

A

Autism Monitoring Tool for the Pediatric Primary Care Clinician

This tool is a form that can be used to document the progress of the autistic child. It provides prompts for each area that requires surveillance, and the options under each heading are ordered from either age-appropriate skills or no symptoms to increasing levels of concern requiring intervention. It is ideal to have this form entered into the electronic health record (EHR) so it can be automatically populated at health supervision visits. Relevant areas covered can be documented, but it is unrealistic to cover all areas at each visit. If possible, this information should be stored in the EHR such that only the items addressed will appear. This information is meant to be a cumulative record of the child's progress that can be used for case management purposes.

Patient name: ______________________________

Date of birth: ______________________________

1. **Developmental assessment**

   Date: ______________________________

   Details: ______________________________

   Findings:

   ☐ Not performed

2. **Neuropsychological testing**

   Date: ______________________________

   Details: ______________________________

   Findings:

   ☐ Not performed

3. **Genetic testing**

   Date: ______________________________

   Details: ______________________________

   Findings:

   ☐ Not performed

4. Neurological history

- ☐ Referral to neurologist ______________________

  Date(s): __________
- ☐ Seizure history
- ☐ Tics

Electroencephalography (EEG):

- ☐ Normal findings
- ☐ Abnormal findings
- ☐ Not performed

5. Hearing and vision history

Hearing screening:

- ☐ Passed in office/audiological examination/brainstem auditory evoked response (BAER)

Vision screening:

- ☐ Passed in office/ophthalmologic examination

  Deaf or hard of hearing: __________ ______________________

  Blind or low vision: __________ ______________________

6. Nutrition history

- ☐ Referral to nutritionist

  Date(s): __________ ______________________
- ☐ Well-balanced diet
- ☐ Feeds self
- ☐ Eats on a schedule
- ☐ Limited repertoire
- ☐ Fed by parent
- ☐ Limited textures
- ☐ Snacks often
- ☐ Holds food in cheeks
- ☐ Gags
- ☐ Vomits

7. Dental history

- ☐ Brushes teeth
  - ☐ Twice a day
  - ☐ Once a day
- ☐ Does not brush teeth
- ☐ Receives regular dental care
- ☐ Does not receive regular dental care

8. Sleep history

- ☐ Sleeps well/independently/without regular interruption

  ______ hours per 24 hours
- ☐ Naps regularly
- ☐ Does not nap
- ☐ Difficulty falling asleep
- ☐ Bed refusal
- ☐ Co-sleeps with parent
- ☐ Night wakening
- ☐ Snores
- ☐ Sleep apnea/gasps
- ☐ Grinds teeth
- ☐ Hard to wake in the morning
- ☐ Falls asleep during day

9. Elimination history

- ☐ Referral to gastroenterologist

  Date(s): __________ ______________________
- ☐ Normal stools
- ☐ Dry at night
- ☐ Toilet trained
  - ☐ Completely
  - ☐ Partially
  - ☐ Only for urine
- ☐ Not toilet trained
- ☐ Bedwetting

- ☐ Abdominal pain
- ☐ Diarrhea
- ☐ Constipation

10. Constipation details (if relevant)

- ☐ No constipation

Constipation symptoms:

- ☐ <3 stools per week
- ☐ Excessive stool retention
- ☐ Painful stools
- ☐ Hard stools
- ☐ Large-diameter stools
- ☐ Fecal incontinence
- ☐ Poor weight gain
- ☐ Blood in stool
- ☐ Lumbosacral tuft or dimple
- ☐ Delayed passage of meconium
- ☐ Vomiting

11. Constipation treatments

- ☐ None
- ☐ Polyethylene glycol 3350
- ☐ Milk of magnesia
- ☐ High-fiber diet
- ☐ Suppository
- ☐ Stool softener
- ☐ Enema
- ☐ Behavioral interventions

Details: ________________________

12. Activities of daily living (ADLs)

- ☐ Age appropriate

Dresses:

- ☐ Independent
- ☐ Needs assistance
- ☐ Dependent

Brushes teeth:

- ☐ Independent
- ☐ Needs assistance
- ☐ Dependent

Maintains hygiene:

- ☐ Independent
- ☐ Needs assistance
- ☐ Dependent

Cares for belongings:

- ☐ Independent
- ☐ Needs assistance
- ☐ Dependent

Follows routines:

- ☐ Independent
- ☐ Needs assistance
- ☐ Dependent

Other ADLs relevant to age (eg, reading bus schedule, riding public transportation, washing laundry, doing dishes, cooking):

____

____

13. Responsibilities

- ☐ Does chores

Homework:

- ☐ Independent
- ☐ Needs assistance
- ☐ Dependent

14. Expressive language

- ☐ Age appropriate
- ☐ Uses words to request
- ☐ Responds to "wh" (what, where, why, when, and who) questions
- ☐ Shares thoughts/ideas
- ☐ Stays on topic, has conversational exchange
- ☐ Tells stories

Speech progress:

- ☐ Emerging
- ☐ Unchanged
- ☐ Improving

Current level:

- ☐ Babbling
- ☐ Jargon
- ☐ Few words
- ☐ Many words

- ☐ Uses only sign language
- ☐ Uses Picture Exchange Communication System
- ☐ Uses augmentative and alternative communication device
- ☐ Self-directed/speaks using self-directed topics rather than responding to others' topics
- ☐ Delayed speech
- ☐ Echolalia
- ☐ Apraxia
- ☐ Nonverbal

15. Receptive language

- ☐ Age appropriate
- ☐ Understands "wh" (what, where, when, why, and who) questions
- ☐ Responds back and forth
- ☐ Understands stories
- ☐ Points to named item
- ☐ Responds to name/familiar requests/variety of requests
- ☐ Does not understand stories
- ☐ Does not understand "wh" (what, where, when, why, and who) questions
- ☐ Does not respond to words
- ☐ Does not respond to name

16. Motor development

Fine motor:

- ☐ Age appropriate
- ☐ Delayed

Gross motor:

- ☐ Age appropriate
- ☐ Delayed

- ☐ Hypotonia
- ☐ Motor planning difficulties
- ☐ Poor coordination
- ☐ Struggles with handwriting

17. Play

- ☐ Takes turns
- ☐ Engages in imaginative play
- ☐ Involved in sports
- ☐ Enters group activities
- ☐ Concrete play: blocks, puzzles, arranging, building
- ☐ Spinning, lining up
- ☐ Throws objects
- ☐ Mouths objects
- ☐ Bangs objects

18. Social skills

- ☐ Has close friends
- ☐ Plays collaboratively with peers
- ☐ Approaches others
- ☐ Initiates play with others
- ☐ Interacts with peers
- ☐ Plays alone
- ☐ Struggles to read cues
- ☐ Aversive reaction to peers

19. Behavior

- ☐ No concerns
- ☐ Anxiety
- ☐ Repetitive behaviors, rituals
- ☐ Irritability
- ☐ Often dysregulated
- ☐ Self-injurious behavior
- ☐ Aggression
- ☐ Asks repetitive questions
- ☐ Struggles with transitions
- ☐ Repetitive movements
- ☐ Intensely preoccupied with own interests
- ☐ Insistent on having things a certain way

20. Attention and activity

- ☐ Good attention span
- ☐ High degree of self-control
- ☐ Stays seated in class
- ☐ Completes tasks consistently
- ☐ Works independently on homework
- ☐ Inattention
- ☐ Easily distracted
- ☐ Fidgets
- ☐ Always moving/active
- ☐ Impulsivity
- ☐ Needs support to complete tasks
- ☐ Disruptive behaviors (to their functioning or others' space)
- ☐ Recent Vanderbilt Assessment Scales:

  Date(s): ____________________
  ____

  Results: ____________________
  ____

21. School services

School placement:

- ☐ Private
- ☐ Special education
- ☐ General education
- ☐ Mixed

- ☐ Applied behavior analysis (ABA)
- ☐ Speech therapy
- ☐ Deaf or hard of hearing specialist (D/HH teacher)
- ☐ Visual impairment specialist (TVI: teacher of students with visual impairments)
- ☐ Augmentative and alternative communication
- ☐ Occupational therapy
- ☐ Physical therapy
- ☐ Feeding therapy
- ☐ Developmental-behavioral pediatrics
- ☐ Psychology
- ☐ Psychiatry
- ☐ Other services: ____________________
  ____

22. Academics

- ☐ Grade level
- ☐ Advanced
- ☐ Areas of concern: ____________________
  ____

23. Special education services

- ☐ Individualized education program (IEP)
- ☐ 504 plan
- ☐ School behavioral intervention plan (BIP)

- ☐ Functional behavioral assessment (FBA)

  Date(s): ______________

  ____

24. Medicaid waiver

Date discussed: ______________

Materials given: ______________

Obtained: ______________

25. Medication (Refer to medication list.)

- ☐ Medication notes
- ☐ Behavioral health medication

26. Safety

- ☐ Wears medical ID
- ☐ Elopement risk
- ☐ Drowning risk
- ☐ GPS tracker device/registered with police department
- ☐ Home safety plan

27. Family history; social drivers of health

- ☐ No concerns
- ☐ Housing insecurity
- ☐ Food insecurity
- ☐ Unemployment
- ☐ Violence
- ☐ Family discord
- ☐ Social supports
- ☐ Mental health condition
- ☐ Loss: divorce, death, family members moving away

28. Strengths

List child's areas of strength:

____

____

29. Goals

- ☐ Academic: ______________
- ☐ Communication: ______________
- ☐ Self-regulation: ______________
- ☐ Behavioral: ______________
- ☐ Sensory processing: ______________
- ☐ Social: ______________
- ☐ Motor skills: ______________
- ☐ Constipation management: ______________
- ☐ Feeding behaviors: ______________
- ☐ Activities of daily living (ADLs): ______________
- ☐ Resources/referrals shared with family: ______________

Created by Polly Panitz, MD, and Amy Pierce, MD.

APPENDIX

B

Parent Handout: What Is Autism and How Do I Know if My Preschool-Aged Child Is on the Spectrum?

1. What is autism and how does it present in early development?

Autism describes a variety of atypical developmental characteristics that tend to be recognizable between 14 and 36 months of age. Children on the autism spectrum may have difficulties in social engagement, communication (use of gesture and use of language), and sensory processing, as well as restricted and repetitive behaviors and interests or ritualistic behaviors. Children on the spectrum may not display ease with back-and-forth social interaction, relationship building, and meeting the demands of everyday life. Many children on the spectrum have remarkable strengths and talents and loving relationships. Despite the concerns at diagnosis, many children respond to early intervention and make significant developmental gains. It is important that parents of children on the spectrum seek professional guidance to create a comprehensive treatment plan that is specific to autism and the needs of the child and family. Talk with your child's pediatric clinician and enroll your child in early intervention services as soon as possible. Waiting to get professional help may lead to missed opportunities for improvement. It is helpful to know the following information about autism:

- Children are born on the spectrum, but autism characteristics are not reliably recognizable until the age at which children are expected to interact and communicate with others, usually around their second birthday.
- There may be early signs of autism, but it cannot be reliably diagnosed before 14 to 16 months of age and about half of those diagnosed are not identified until their third birthday.
- For some children, concerns for an autism diagnosis may be raised later in life, when they have difficulties in academic and social settings.
- Autism is relatively common; it occurs in about 1 out of 31 children and is more common in boys.
- Autism in girls may go undetected more often because of girls' ability to learn ways to fit in with their peers.

- An autism diagnosis is assigned after a series of formalized behavioral observations are made by a professional with an MD/DO or PhD/PsyD degree. It is defined by the child meeting a specific set of behavioral characteristics. The professional will use questionnaires and tests that differentiate typical development from atypical development. They will evaluate other possible contributors to developmental delay such as expressive language disorder, intellectual disability, and abnormal genetics. Genetic conditions such as Down syndrome or fragile X syndrome are likely to affect a child's developmental course. The features of these syndromes may appear in addition to the diagnosis of autism, independent of autism, or as features that require careful assessment to differentiate from autism.
- The primary challenges for young children on the spectrum are delays in social engagement and interaction (refer to the Resources on Joint Attention and Autism section at the end of this handout).
- The skills in social engagement and interaction are referred to as *skills of joint attention*. The development of these skills creates a foundation for learning, communication, play, and engagement with others. The presence of joint attention is associated with successful communication skills later in life, as joint attention is used to share, communicate, and initiate interaction with others.
- Joint attention develops as a child explores their world and learns to share this attention with caregivers. The child watches as the adult uses eye contact and gaze, pointing, and words to share and communicate. The child follows and imitates the parent and then learns to use these skills on their own as they explore their world. They learn to coordinate eye gaze and use gesture (pointing) to share their interest in something with another person. By 14 months of age, the child will shift eye gaze from object to parent and use pointing and other forms of gesture along with vocalizations to communicate effectively.

2. What are the early signs of autism?

Many of the early signs of autism can be seen briefly in typically developing children at various points in development and may have no significance **if** they exist alone. In autism, the features of concern are continual and widespread and become more impactful to the child. The early signs of autism may include

- Lack of spontaneous sharing of pleasure and interests
- Decreased eye contact for communicating with others (A child may look at others but without intent to communicate.)
- Lack of response to being called
- Not sharing interests with others
- Unusual cadence of language

- Lack of awareness of others
- Absence of babbling
- Uses parent's hand or body as a guiding tool to indicate their requests, rather than uses forms of communication
- Does not play with toys, but uses them in an atypical or repetitive fashion (flips over and spins wheels, opens toys up, lines them up, moves them from place to place, gathers and drops, throws, or categorizes in a systematic way)
- Has excessively strong interests, such as in letters, numbers, colors, or specific videos, without the typical variety seen in peers
- Loses skills that were previously present
- Talks, sings, or babbles to self
- Repetitive movements or use of objects—for example, toe walking or flicking things
- Restricted and repetitive rituals—for example, turning on and off lights or other electric operations, opening and closing doors, or staring at something out of the corner of their eye, perhaps while in an unusual position
- Uses words to mimic others or only to label pictures or objects rather than uses words to call, interact, or make requests of others
- Has excessive tantrums, is hard to comfort
- Has unusual sensory difficulties, such as fear/panic with everyday sounds, textures, or experiences—for example, toilets flushing, vacuum cleaners, or specific foods or clothing
- Low muscle tone or poor motor coordination

3. How can I support my child?

Children learn to explore relationships and they develop the skills of joint attention through play. During play, they develop ideas, learn to think about ideas, and engage and communicate with others. You can teach your child skills of social engagement and turn taking through play! Here are steps you can take to help your child learn these skills.

Play with your child! Here are some therapeutic maneuvers that will motivate your child to play with you and to interact and develop the skills of joint attention they may lack. The aim of this type of intervention is to teach your child to **attend to others, develop relationships, learn to problem-solve, and develop the functional use of language.** Since the core feature of autism is a delay in social engagement, working on these skills first will ensure the strongest foundation for growth.

1. **Encourage eye contact and face-to-face interaction.** Position yourself at your child's eye level, face-to-face. Make yourself animated and expressive, use animated inflections in your voice, and use singing or nursery rhymes to motivate your child to attend to you. Change your actions, inflections, and level of expression to those that effectively gain your child's attention; some children can be overwhelmed when a parent is animated, expressive, and very playful, while others find this appealing. You may need to raise or lower your volume or the dynamic nature of your movements and responses to match the needs of your child. Pay attention to what works with *your* child.
2. **Remove distractions.** Turn off screens and audio, put away distracting toys, such as electronic toys or toys or items your child tends to focus on intensively.
3. **Ensure your child's preferred toys are out of reach.** Place preferred toys out of the child's reach or inside clear containers so they need you to obtain them and so you can work on the child's requesting behaviors.
4. **Find enticing toys for play.** Use toys that will encourage your child to engage, such as bubbles, balloons, windup toys, balls, or cars for passing back and forth, to maximize your success. Activate or pass the toy to get your child's attention, then hold the object and **wait** to encourage your child to either look at you or try to ask for more. If your child is playing in a repetitive fashion, such as moving a car back and forth, playfully block their movement or make a car crash into another object in an attempt to turn the action into an interaction with **you**! If they do not look up, make some movement or say something like "Ready, set, go!" or "Here we go!" in an animated way to motivate your child to look at you. Sometimes holding the toy near your face will encourage more face-to-face interaction. (Please note that you cannot always achieve true eye contact, but the goal is to encourage the child to look at their play partner so they can gain information from your emotional expression during an interaction.)
5. **Allow for extra time.** When playing with your child or encouraging your child to make requests, allow extra time for your child to respond or use the skills they have. Often we direct and fill in responses too quickly for the child without giving them an opportunity to respond. Some children will need extra time to show their skills. When you are playing, **pause and allow your child the time** to take the next step or look at you.
6. **Recognize your child's sensory needs.** Avoid triggers that overwhelm your child and use types of play that are pleasurable, interesting, and calming for your child. Some sounds, types of touch, smell, movement, or actions can be aversive to your child, while others can have a positive effect; observe and take notes about how different forms of sensory input affect your child.

7. **Observe how your child indicates what they want and give them time to look back at you and use gestures or vocalizations.** If your child moves directly toward the object or pulls you toward it, make certain that desirable items (food and preferred toys) are out of reach to create opportunities for your child to learn to ask with gesture and use eye contact and vocalization. Model a request using simple words 1 to 2 at a time ("Want cookie" or "Give milk") and simple gestures (pointing) and put yourself into a place where your child is more likely to be able to look at you. Practice this type of requesting often. Reinforce it by giving the child what they seek.

8. **Imitate your child's actions and use simple vocalizations.** To make the play about taking turns, teaching language, and being social, get down to your child's level and mimic their actions, using simple words and vocalizations. Having 2 of each toy will avoid any resistance to sharing. Have 2 drums and enjoy imitating your child banging on the drums, then work toward turn taking in this activity. Introduce a relevant word or phrase such as "drum" or "bang" or "My turn/Your turn," model the use of the word, and **wait** for your child to imitate.

9. **Respond to your child's attempts to communicate.** Respond with praise, such as "Wow, great job!" Reinforce all your child's attempts to communicate with an enthusiastic comment or response that will build on their request or comment. Respond in a way that relates to what you think they are saying ("Oh, you want drum"). Your response can teach your child a new word or gesture.

10. **Use some simple repetitive phrases to encourage communication and attention.** Using phrases such as "Ready, set, go" when doing something desirable such as chasing, tickling, or swinging can encourage your child to communicate and remain engaged. As a next step, only say "Ready, set" and pause to encourage your child to fill in "go." Become animated as you both say "go" to encourage eye contact and engagement.

11. **Use simple 1- to 2-word phrases to teach basic communication and practice often.** Teach simple requests such as "Open," "Go," or "Eat" when your child clearly wants an activity. Try teaching a sign for this at first as your child is learning to imitate verbally. Create opportunities to teach these words often while playing throughout the day. Use purposeful and specific words, rather than more generalized words, such as "Please" or "More," that the child may use for any request.

12. **Sing songs and nursery rhymes to encourage vocal imitation and turn taking.** Once your child has learned lines from a song or nursery rhyme, pause when reciting to let them fill in the missing word. Always remember to position yourself to encourage face-to-face interaction. Sitting at a small table can help with this.

13 **Play games involving physical interaction that are motivating, such as chase, tickling, or swinging the child in your arms.** Use the same word and action each time and pause before continuing to encourage your child to make a request and look at you. Model for them to "Tickle" or "Push" before continuing to find motivating opportunities for the child to ask for more of the activity.

14 **Work on modeling pointing for your child.** When they see preferred pictures in books or toys, point to them. Next, model using pointing when things are farther away. Incorporate this into daily play to encourage your child to imitate the use of pointing.

15 **Include your child's interests in your play and turn them into a game.** Playing games such as hiding, peekaboo, or back-and-forth passing can be particularly motivating. Bring the play into the shared space between you so you and your child are face-to-face. Follow your child's lead in play and find opportunities for teaching within this play (new vocabulary or requests). Remember that sometimes simply imitating what your child prefers to do can gain their attention and lead to interaction.

16 **Respond to your child's vocalizations as if they are intentional.** If they say "crayon," grab a crayon and color.

17 **Model for your child what you want the response to be.** Some children will echo what the parent has said rather than respond and thereby reverse pronouns. You may ask, "Do you want a cookie?" and the child may affirm or respond, "You want a cookie." You will need to model the appropriate use of first-person pronouns when a child is making a request, such as "I want a cookie" as you get a cookie for your child.

18 **Make book reading fun!** Allow the child to turn the pages, add song or action to the story, act out the story with objects, or add words or paraphrase to motivate their interest.

19 **Introduce new skills when you have success with an interaction.** If you are happily playing by passing a ball back and forth, continue to build on that positive engagement. For example, model using a relevant word ("go" or "ball") as you pass the ball and slow down the pace of the game to give your child time to imitate or attempt to imitate, look up at you, and ask for the ball.

20 **Use fewer words and follow through more.** Attempt to avoid the pitfall of asking your child excessive questions ("What is this?") or always telling them what to do. As adults, we tend to ask our children to perform often. This can be exhausting or aversive to some children. Rather, attempt to create opportunities that are interesting to your child and that encourage them to use their language. Give them the smallest prompt necessary and give them time to show their skills. For instance, go to the door, put your hand on the handle, wait until they look up at you, and then wave or model "Goodbye" rather than tell them to say it. Reward them with a warm smile and response.

21. **Build on your child's play by taking it to the next step.** If your child builds a tower of blocks, turn it into a house and put people inside or make the blocks talk or interact. This will model how to add a level of symbolic or pretend play when a child demonstrates only the concrete use of objects (to build).

Resources on Joint Attention and Autism

- Autism Navigator ASD Video Glossary (https://autismnavigator.com/asd-video-glossary): video examples of joint attention and other early signs of autism compared to typical development in children of the same age
- *An Early Start for Your Child with Autism: Using Everyday Activities to Help Kids Connect, Communicate, and Learn* by Sally J. Rogers, PhD; Geraldine Dawson, PhD; and Laurie A. Vismara, PhD: a parent guide providing teaching tools and strategies based on the Early Start Denver Model (ESDM)
- The Hanen Centre (www.hanen.org/home): online courses and handouts for parents on fostering joint attention, play, communication, and early literacy
- Help is in Your Hands (www.helpisinyourhands.org): free parent video series on autism therapy for the young child from the ESDM, a research-based group providing a curriculum for teaching young children on the autism spectrum
- *How to Help Your Child With Joint Attention* by Bryony Rust, speech pathologist (www.youtube.com/watch?v=iN09CEMmKIQ): video about joint attention with simple suggestions to support it
- *More Than Words: A Parent's Guide to Building Interaction and Language Skills for Children with Autism Spectrum Disorder or Social Communication Difficulties,* Second Edition, by Fern Sussman: a guide for parents to teach play, social engagement, and conversational exchange

APPENDIX

C

Sample Intake Questionnaire

(To be completed by the parent[s] before an appointment)

1. GENERAL INFORMATION

Date: ______________________

Child's Name: ______________________

Date of Birth: ______________________

Age: ______________________

Person/people completing questionnaire:

Relationship to child:

a. What questions do you have about your child today?

____

____

____

b. What are your child's strengths? Please describe:

____

____

____

c. What are your goals for this evaluation?

____

____

____

d. How long have you had these concerns?

____

____

____

e. Was there anything that brought these concerns on?

____

____

____

f. What have you tried that has been been successful?

______

______

______

g. What have you tried that has not been successful?

______

______

______

h. In what contexts do these concerns arise?

- ☐ Home
- ☐ School
- ☐ Other; please describe: ______

______

______

i. Name of school/child care facility: ______

j. Does your child have any of the following plans in place?

- ☐ Individualized education program (IEP)
- ☐ Individualized family service plan (IFSP)
- ☐ Section 504 plan

k. Have they been evaluated by early intervention or special education service professionals?

☐ Yes ☐ No

Please explain: ______

______

______

l. List all services your child receives: ______

______

______

2. BIRTH HISTORY

Which number pregnancy was this child? ______

Prior pregnancies:

Check the relevant option(s) and list the number.

- ☐ Terminations? If yes, how many? ______
- ☐ Miscarriages? If yes, how many? ______
- ☐ Live births? If yes, how many? ______

Was this child born early?

- ☐ If yes, how early? ____________
- ☐ No

Birth weight: ____________ Apgar score (if known): ____________

- ☐ Vaginal birth?
- ☐ Cesarean birth? Reason: ____________

Were there any challenges with the pregnancy? **PLEASE CHECK ALL THAT ARE RELEVANT.**

- ☐ Hospitalizations
- ☐ History of infertility
- ☐ Bleeding
- ☐ Medications; please describe: ____________

____

- ☐ Alcohol use
- ☐ Cigarette smoking/vaping
- ☐ Other drug use (eg, cannabis, hallucinogen)
- ☐ Complications such as toxemia, diabetes, injuries/accidents, or infections; please describe: ____________

____

Was this child kept in the special care nursery? ☐ Yes ☐ No

If yes, please explain: ____________

____

Home from the hospital in how many days? ____________

Challenges in the first month after birth? ☐ Yes ☐ No

If yes, please explain: ____________

____

Describe your child as an infant, including any challenges: ____________

____

Check any that apply to your child in the first months after birth.

- ☐ Irritability; please describe: ____________

____

- ☐ Difficult to arouse; please describe: ____________

____

- ☐ Poor weight gain/feeding; please describe: ____________

____

Newborn feeding; please describe: ____________________

____

☐ Breastfed only — How long? ____________________

☐ Bottle-fed only — How long? ____________________

☐ Both breastfed and bottle-fed — How long? ____________________

3. MEDICAL HISTORY

Has your child had any of the following conditions? **PLEASE CHECK ALL THAT APPLY.**

☐ Heart disease

☐ Irregular heart rate

☐ Fainting

☐ Chest pain

☐ Frequent illnesses; please describe: ____________________

____

☐ Surgical procedures; please describe: ____________________

____

☐ Hospitalizations; please describe: ____________________

____

☐ Head injuries/accidents; please describe: ____________________

____

☐ Your child's behavior changes during an illness: ☐ Loses skills? ☐ Gains skills?

Please describe: ____________________

____

Past medical concerns/conditions: ____________________

____

____

Present medical concerns/conditions: ____________________

____

____

Specialists your child has seen; please include the reason:

a. ____________________

____

b. ____________________

____

c. ____

____

d. ____

____

Has your child had a formal hearing test? ☐ Yes ☐ No

If yes, where? ____

Do they wear glasses? ☐ Yes ☐ No

If yes, why? ____

____

4. MEDICATIONS/ALLERGIES

Medications: ____

____

Nutritional or other treatments: ____

____

Confirmed allergies: ____

____

Food intolerances/suspected allergies: ____

____

5. DEVELOPMENTAL HISTORY

Please list the age at which the following milestones were first seen:

AGE	MILESTONE
	First smile
	Babbled, repeated consonant sounds like "mama" or "baba"
	Weaned off breast/bottle
	Sat alone
	Walked independently
	Spoke first meaningful words to ask for things or call parents
	Put words together
	Spoke 2- to 3-word sentences
	Fed self with spoon/fork
	Able to dress self

AGE	MILESTONE
	Able to separate from parent
	Potty trained
	Slept through the night
	Pointed to get someone's attention

Skills of independence:

Toileting: Urinates in diaper ☐ or toilet ☐ Has bowel movement in diaper ☐ or toilet ☐

Diarrhea: ☐ Yes ☐ No Constipation: ☐ Yes ☐ No Has accidents: ☐ Yes ☐ No

Can your child dress independently? ☐ Yes ☐ No Undress? ☐ Yes ☐ No

Handle zippers? ☐ Yes ☐ No Put on shoes? ☐ Yes ☐ No

Help with chores? ☐ Yes ☐ No

Help with cleanup? ☐ Yes ☐ No

PLEASE CHECK ALL THAT APPLY TO YOUR CHILD PRESENTLY.				
Behavioral Trait	**Rarely**	**Occasionally**	**Often**	**Unable to Comment**
Irritability	☐	☐	☐	☐
Difficult to comfort	☐	☐	☐	☐
Difficulty with frustration	☐	☐	☐	☐
Difficulty with transitions	☐	☐	☐	☐
Difficulty with new people	☐	☐	☐	☐
Frequently ill	☐	☐	☐	☐
Frequently tired	☐	☐	☐	☐
Concerned about neatness or cleanliness	☐	☐	☐	☐
Resists cuddling	☐	☐	☐	☐
Resists getting touched, wearing clothing, or touching certain textures—for example, food, liquids, or sticky things	☐	☐	☐	☐
Startles easily with sounds	☐	☐	☐	☐
Becomes overexcited in busy settings	☐	☐	☐	☐
Puts objects into mouth	☐	☐	☐	☐
Bullies	☐	☐	☐	☐
Seems fearless	☐	☐	☐	☐
Has few friends	☐	☐	☐	☐
Seems sad, unhappy, or anxious	☐	☐	☐	☐
Has difficulty with separation	☐	☐	☐	☐

PLEASE CHECK ALL THAT APPLY TO YOUR CHILD PRESENTLY.				
Behavioral Trait	**Rarely**	**Occasionally**	**Often**	**Unable to Comment**
Is not liked by other children	☐	☐	☐	☐
Seems unaware of other children	☐	☐	☐	☐
Has trouble with changes in routine	☐	☐	☐	☐
Asks for help too frequently	☐	☐	☐	☐
Is always active	☐	☐	☐	☐
Has intense moods	☐	☐	☐	☐
Is easily distracted	☐	☐	☐	☐
Often does not respond to others	☐	☐	☐	☐
Has excessive routines/rituals	☐	☐	☐	☐
Makes eye contact	☐	☐	☐	☐
Uses single words	☐	☐	☐	☐
Uses phrases	☐	☐	☐	☐
Uses sentences	☐	☐	☐	☐
Points to things	☐	☐	☐	☐
Takes turns speaking	☐	☐	☐	☐
Uses words to ask	☐	☐	☐	☐
Pulls a person when they want something	☐	☐	☐	☐
Uses pronouns	☐	☐	☐	☐
Responds to requests	☐	☐	☐	☐
Responds to being called	☐	☐	☐	☐
Responds when you try to get their attention by pointing to something	☐	☐	☐	☐
Points on request	☐	☐	☐	☐
Echoes what others say	☐	☐	☐	☐
Repeats language from TV	☐	☐	☐	☐
Can follow 1- or 2-step instructions	☐	☐	☐	☐
Uses words to ask for things	☐	☐	☐	☐
Answers yes/no questions	☐	☐	☐	☐
Answers "wh" (what, where, why, when, and who) questions	☐	☐	☐	☐
Asks for help	☐	☐	☐	☐
Has focused interests	☐	☐	☐	☐
Tells a story	☐	☐	☐	☐

PLEASE CHECK ALL THAT APPLY TO YOUR CHILD PRESENTLY.				
Behavioral Trait	**Rarely**	**Occasionally**	**Often**	**Unable to Comment**
Reads some words	☐	☐	☐	☐
Reads fluently	☐	☐	☐	☐
Identifies numbers	☐	☐	☐	☐
Identifies letters	☐	☐	☐	☐
Identifies shapes	☐	☐	☐	☐

Approximate vocabulary size: ______________________________

6. SPECIFIC BEHAVIORAL CHALLENGES

Check all areas of struggle that apply and describe as indicated.

☐ Mealtime challenges, such as throwing food, staying seated, or coming to the table?

If yes, please describe: ______________________________

____

____

☐ Excessive tantrums?

If yes, please list frequency, duration, and common triggers: ______________________________

____

____

☐ Struggles to engage with other children (turn taking, sharing, initiating interactions with peers, and sustaining interactions with peers)?

If yes, please describe: ______________________________

____

____

☐ Repetitive behaviors—for example, hand flapping, spinning, opening/closing doors, head banging, or turning lights on and off?

If yes, please describe: ______________________________

____

____

☐ Lines up or arranges objects rather than plays with them?

If yes, please describe: ______________________________

____

☐ Aggressive behavior?

If yes, please describe: ______________________________

☐ Self-injurious behavior—for example, bangs head or hits, bites, or scratches self?

If yes, please describe: ______________________________

☐ Struggles to follow instructions?

If yes, please describe: ______________________________

☐ Other: ______________________________

7. PLAY BEHAVIORS: Check all that are relevant to your child.

Does your child:

☐ Play with toys as expected?

☐ Engage in pretend play with ideas, such as feeding a stuffed animal, putting a doll to sleep, having their play cars involved in going somewhere, or having their play figures interact or have dialogue?

☐ Seek out others to play?

☐ Have close friends?

☐ Act in pretend roles in play with others, such as becoming a character during play?

☐ Seem happy to play alone?

8. SLEEP HISTORY

YES	NO	DOES YOUR CHILD:
		Wake during the night?
		Have trouble with bedtime routine?
		Struggle to fall asleep alone?
		Snore or gasp for breath during sleep?
		Wake early?
		Seem sleepy or fall asleep during the day?

No. of hours of sleep per day: ________

9. DIET HISTORY

How many ounces of each does your child drink daily? _______ water _______ milk

_______ juice _______ soda

Your child drinks from: ☐ Open cup ☐ Sippy cup ☐ Straw ☐ Bottle

No. of servings of dairy per day: ____________________

Does your child feed themselves? ☐ Yes ☐ No

Do adults feed your child? ☐ Yes ☐ No

Does your child eat a limited variety of foods? ☐ Yes ☐ No

Do they put excessive amounts of food into their mouth? ☐ Yes ☐ No

Do they gag or vomit often when eating? ☐ Yes ☐ No

List your child's favorite foods: ____________________

Please describe the typical foods your child eats for each meal.

Breakfast: ____________________

Lunch: ____________________

Dinner: ____________________

Snacks: ____________________

10. FAMILY HISTORY

Who lives in the child's primary home? Include the parent(s).

NAME	AGE	RELATIONSHIP
a.		
b.		
c.		
d.		
e.		
f.		

Does the child have a secondary home? ☐ Yes ☐ No

Who lives in the secondary home?

a. ______________________ b. ______________________

c. ______________________ d. ______________________

e. ______________________ f. ______________________

PARENTS

☐ Married ☐ Divorced ☐ Separated

☐ Never married ☐ Living together ☐ Living separately

☐ Parent working out of state, such as for a military deployment; if yes, please describe:

____

Biological father's highest level of education: ______________________

Biological father's occupation: ______________________

Biological mother's highest level of education: ______________________

Biological mother's occupation: ______________________

Language(s) spoken at home:

Primary: ______________________ Other: ______________________

Are you the biological parent(s) of this child? ☐ Yes ☐ No

If not, please share history: ______________________

____

Other family members regularly involved with child: ______________________

____

Other adults regularly involved with child: ______________________

____

Does your child have a babysitter? ☐ Yes ☐ No

If yes, please indicate the setting:

☐ In your home ☐ In a child care facility ☐ Through in-home child care

What are their observations/concerns? ______________________

____

____

Have any family members had the following conditions? Check all that apply, indicate the family member, and provide relevant descriptions.

CHECK IF APPLICABLE.		FAMILY MEMBER	DESCRIPTION
Hyperactivity or attention-deficit/hyperactivity disorder	☐		
Trouble learning in school/learning disability	☐		
Delayed language	☐		
Delayed/awkward social skills	☐		
Autism	☐		
Seizures	☐		
Behavioral challenges	☐		
Depression	☐		
Alcohol or drug use	☐		
Anxiety, bipolar disorder, schizophrenia	☐		
Heart disease/cardiac death	☐		
Irregular heart rhythm	☐		
Fainting spells	☐		
Chronic medical issues	☐		
Cancer	☐		
Parents related	☐		
Infertility	☐		
Early menopause	☐		
Chronic neurological conditions	☐		

Has this child been exposed to any stressful events such as bullying, family discord/dispute, homelessness, food insecurity, violence, inappropriate touch or abuse, or the death of a loved one? ☐ Yes ☐ No

If yes, please describe: ______________________________

____

____

Other comments: ______________________________

____

____

____

____

____

APPENDIX

D

Diagnostic Criteria for Electronic Health Record Documentation

This checklist is derived from the *Diagnostic and Statistical Manual of Mental Disorders, Fifth Edition, Text Revision* (*DSM-5-TR*) diagnostic criteria and provides a list of clinical signs grouped under the specific diagnostic criteria categories. It is suggested to be used as saved text in the electronic health record to streamline documentation of the diagnostic features of autism spectrum disorder (ASD). The list is long and inclusive, and the options can be included or eliminated as is relevant to the particular child.

After a thorough review of the child's medical, developmental, social, and family history, the clinician performed a physical examination with attention to the neurological examination, growth parameters, and potential dysmorphic features and made developmental and structured behavioral observations. It is found that the child demonstrates significant and persistent difficulties in social communication and interaction across multiple contexts as well as restricted and repetitive patterns of behaviors, interests, and/or activities. Thus, the child meets *DSM-5-TR* criteria for a diagnosis of ASD. The following relevant findings were observed in examinations today as denoted by a checkmark:

1. **Challenges in social communication and interaction (must have findings in all 3 categories):**

______ a. Delays in social reciprocity: Limited showing, directing attention, and sharing of enjoyment; does not initiate interactions or respond consistently to the social bids of others; inconsistent response to name; communication is focused on specific interests.

______ b. Atypical nonverbal social behavior: Inconsistent or atypical eye gaze; limited pointing, facial expression, or gesture use; uses the bodies of others as a tool; cannot communicate needs or wants.

______ c. Difficulties in maintaining relationships: Limited interest in peer play, limited participation in interactive games, struggles with basic social/safety rules, limited imitative and pretend play.

2. Restricted and repetitive patterns of behaviors and interests (must have characteristics within 2 of the 4 categories):

_______ a. Stereotypical, repetitive, idiosyncratic speech, use of objects, or motor movements: Echolalia; scripting; pronoun reversal; atypical jargoning (not purposeful speech); body, hand, or finger mannerisms (eg, hand flapping, tensing, finger flicking, inspecting, rocking, clapping, toe walking, facial grimacing); repetitive use of objects (lining them up, organizing, moving back and forth, spinning, dropping, throwing, or showing interest in parts of objects).

_______ b. Excessive adherence to routines: Performs activities in exact sequence or manner, becomes distressed when a routine is changed, repeats specific sequences in play, insists on sameness.

_______ c. Atypical sensory behavior: Visual inspection, noise sensitivity, atypical pain threshold or hyperfocus on physical stimulation, sensory aversions (eg, smells, foods, textures, touch), sensory-seeking experiences.

_______ d. Focused interests: Requiring certain objects to always be present, unusual interests (eg, vacuums, shiny objects, fans, doors), intense focal interests.

3. It was determined by this assessment today that the following circumstances are true:

_______ a. Symptoms were present in the early developmental period (usually by ages 2–3 years) or became apparent when social demands exceeded capacities.

_______ b. Symptoms result in clinically significant difficulty in social, occupational, or other functional domains.

_______ c. Symptoms are not attributed to intellectual disability (ID) (or global developmental delay).

4. Specify if the following circumstances are true:

_______ a. Accompanying ID

_______ b. Accompanying language disorder

5. Severity level specified as follows:

_______ Level 3: Severe difficulties in both verbal and nonverbal social communication skills result in severe interference with functioning and extreme inflexibility of behavior that require very substantial support.

_______ Level 2: Significant challenges in both verbal and nonverbal social communication skills result in interference with functioning, noted while support is in place, and inflexibility of behavior, interfering with everyday experiences, that require substantial support.

_______ Level 1: Difficulties in social communication exist without supports in place and inflexibility of behavior causes significant interference with functioning and requires support.

Derived from Autism spectrum disorder. In: American Psychiatric Association. *Diagnostic and Statistical Manual of Mental Disorders.* 5th ed text rev. American Psychiatric Association; 2022:56–68.

APPENDIX

E

Diagnostic Criteria Checklist With Developmental Anchors

This checklist is based on the *Diagnostic and Statistical Manual of Mental Disorders, Fifth Edition, Text Revision* (*DSM-5-TR*) diagnostic criteria and is a tool for facilitating a diagnosis of autism spectrum disorder in a child. To be of clinical significance, these developmental-behavioral markers must be persistent and pervasive and cause clinically significant difficulty in social, occupational, or other areas of current daily functioning. These features are grouped under the *DSM-5-TR* categories necessary for diagnosis.

Cluster A: Persistent deficits in social communication and social interaction: Deficits and impairment must be present in all 3 symptom domains.

***DSM-5-TR* Symptom**	**Developmental Markers** ***(Mark "O" for "Observed" and "R" for "Reported.")***
____Deficits in social reciprocity	O/R Limited showing, directing attention, sharing of enjoyment/attention with others O/R Does not frequently initiate interactions with others O/R Inconsistent response to social bids of others O/R Inconsistent response to name or attempts to get attention O/R Limited sharing or back-and-forth play O/R Focused language or communication on particular interests
____Atypical nonverbal social behavior	O/R Atypical or inconsistent eye gaze O/R Limited index pointing O/R Limited conventional gesture use (eg, head shaking/nodding, waving, reaching) O/R Limited other gesture use (eg, emphasizing, miming, pretend) O/R Physical direction of others (eg, leading, hand as a tool use) O/R Challenges communicating wants and needs O/R Limited range of directed facial expressions (eg, extremes only)
____Deficits in maintaining relationships	O/R Limited or inconsistent interest in peer interaction and play O/R Limited or inconsistent skills participating in interactive games with siblings/adults O/R Challenges appreciating basic social/safety rules O/R Limited or inconsistent response to approach of novel peers and adults O/R Limited spontaneous initiation of play/interaction O/R Limited imitative and pretend play

Cluster B: Restricted, repetitive patterns of behavior, interests, or activities: Deficits and impairment in 2 of the following 4 domains:

***DSM-5-TR* Symptom**	**Developmental Markers** ***(Mark "O" for "Observed" and "R" for "Reported.")***
____Stereotyped, repetitive, idiosyncratic speech; motor stereotypies; repetitive use of objects	*Speech/language:* O/R Echolalia, scripting O/R Atypical jargoning (undirected speech, peculiar vocalizations) O/R Idiosyncratic speech (pronominal reversal, neologisms) *Motor stereotypies:* O/R Body/hand/finger mannerisms/posturing (eg, hand flapping, tensing, finger/ear flicking, hand/finger inspection, rocking, spinning, repetitive clapping, toe walking, facial grimacing) *Objects:* O/R Repetitive use of objects (eg, lining up, organizing, stacking, spinning, dropping, repeated activation, interest in parts of objects)
____Excessive adherence to nonfunctional routines	O/R Requires activities performed in exact same way (eg, requires caregivers to say things in certain order, motor rituals) O/R Distresses surrounding changing routine (eg, placement of objects in house, change in physical appearance to others, driving route, order of daily activities, food presentation) O/R Carries out specific sequence in play or other activities O/R Insistence on sameness (eg, extreme reaction to changes)
____Atypical sensory behavior (hyposensitivity or hypersensitivity or interest)	O/R Visual interest/inspection O/R Noise sensitivity O/R Atypical pain threshold/strong interest in physical stimulation O/R Sensory aversions (smells, textures, touch, daily routine challenges) O/R Sensory-seeking behavior (sights, smells, mouthing, loud noises, tactile interests)
____Restricted/fixated interests	O/R Requires certain objects to be on their person at all times O/R Focused repetitive play (eg, sorting/stacking/lining up objects) O/R Unusual interests in objects (eg, appliances, fans, mirrors, shiny objects) O/R Intense/rigid focal interests (eg, cars, trains, specific videos, vacuums)

Adapted with permission from Vanderbilt University Medical Center. *DSM-5* checklist with developmental markers. Vanderbilt Kennedy Center. Accessed March 4, 2026. https://vkc.vumc.org.

APPENDIX

F

Parent Resources on Autism

- The Arc (https://thearc.org): A national advocacy organization for individuals with intellectual and developmental disabilities. Provides links for local chapters.
- Autism Navigator (https://autismnavigator.com): An excellent educational resource with a video glossary to illustrate elements that distinguish young children on the autism spectrum from neurotypical children.
- Autism Society (https://autismsociety.org): A website for parents that has many resources, educational materials, and event listings.
- Autism Speaks (www.autismspeaks.org): Includes a wealth of educational materials, specific toolkits on topics, and lists of local resources.
- *Autism Spectrum Disorder: What Every Parent Needs to Know,* 2nd Edition, by Alan I. Rosenblatt, MD, and Paul S. Carbone, MD: A review of autism (diagnosis and care) written for parents.
- *The Complete Guide to Asperger's Syndrome* by Tony Attwood: A thorough review of the developmental processes seen in autism.
- Early Start Denver Model (www.esdm.co): An evidence-based behavioral and developmental curriculum taught in the natural environment to support communication, social engagement, and developmental progress for the young child up to 60 months of age.
- *An Early Start for Your Child with Autism: Using Everyday Activities to Help Kids Connect, Communicate, and Learn* by Sally J. Rogers, PhD; Geraldine Dawson, PhD; and Laurie A. Vismara, PhD: A curriculum for teaching young children on the spectrum. Available as a book.
- HealthyChildren.org, the official American Academy of Pediatrics (AAP) website for parents (www.healthychildren.org/English/health-issues/conditions/Autism/Pages/default.aspx): Autism information for parents, from the AAP.
- Help is in Your Hands (www.helpisinyourhands.org/course/student/dashboard/8585#null): Free teaching tool for parents of preschoolers on the spectrum; requires registration to access.
- *More Than Words: A Parent's Guide to Building Interaction and Language Skills for Children with Autism Spectrum Disorder or Social Communication Difficulties,* Second Edition, and *TalkAbility: People Skills for Verbal Children on the Autism Spectrum—A Guide for Parents* by Fern Sussman: Books for teaching social communication.
- *No More Meltdowns: Positive Strategies for Managing and Preventing Out-of-Control Behavior* by Jed Baker, PhD: A resource for behavioral care and approaches.

- *The Out-of-Sync Child: Recognizing and Coping with Sensory Processing Differences,* Third Edition, by Carol Stock Kranowitz: A book on identifying and working with sensory challenges in children.
- *Overcoming Autism: Finding the Answers, Strategies, and Hope That Can Transform a Child's Life* by Lynn Kern Koegel, PhD, and Claire LaZebnick: An overall guide to autism with resources on behavioral care.
- POAC Autism Services (www.poac.net): National organization of parent-run groups to provide education, advocacy, support, and community.
- Parent resource centers in public schools: Each county will have Community Parent Resource Centers available within publicly funded special education programming to provide education and support to families with children with disabilities.
- Social Thinking (www.socialthinking.com): Social skills curricula and tools developed by Michelle Garcia Winner, MA, CCC-SLP, and Pamela Crooke, PhD, CC-SLP.
- *Solving Executive Function Challenges: Simple Ways to Get Kids with Autism Unstuck and on Target* by Lauren Kenworthy, PhD; Laura Gutermuth Anthony, PhD; Katie Alexander, MS, OTR; Monica Werner, MA; Lynn Cannon, MEd; and Lisa Greenman, JD: An evidence-based curriculum for teaching executive function skills. Written for use by educators and parents to teach behavioral flexibility, goal setting, and organizational skills.
- *The Survival Guide for Kids with Autism Spectrum Disorder (and Their Parents)* by Elizabeth Verdick and Elizabeth Reeve, MD: A child's guide to autism, including an excellent description of autism written for the child.
- Vanderbilt Kennedy Center Treatment and Research Institute for Autism Spectrum Disorders (https://vkc.vumc.org/vkc/triad/home): Resources for families with autistic children.
- The Zones of Regulation by Leah Kuypers, MAEd, OTR/L (https://zonesofregulation.com): An emotional regulation curriculum that teaches the child to recognize their feelings of dysregulation and provides tools for self-regulation. Tools are provided for educators, therapists, and parents.

APPENDIX

G

Sample Letter to Request Evaluation for Special Education Services

This is a letter to request the initiation of evaluation for a suspected developmental delay that is affecting your child's progress. This letter should be sent to the school principal as well as any other professionals at the school involved with your child.

[Date]

[Name of principal]

[School name]

[School address]

RE: [Name of child]

Dear [Name of principal]:

I/We are writing to you to express concern that my/our child has a developmental delay that has a significant negative effect on my/our child's learning. I/we are concerned that my/our child is in need of special education services. As a result, I/we are requesting that the school perform a multidisciplinary team evaluation to include speech and language, psychological, and educational assessments. I/We understand that the team will first need to meet to review my/our child's progress, and I/we request that this meeting occur as soon as possible.

Please send me/us any relevant forms that will need to be completed, and please keep me/us regularly informed of your progress. I/We understand that your response to my/our request is legally mandated and look forward to meeting with the team as soon as possible.

Please respond to this request to confirm its receipt. Thank you for your time and consideration.

Sincerely,

[Your name(s)]

[Your legal role(s)]

[Your contact information]

INDEX

Page numbers followed by *f*, *b*, and *t* indicate figures, boxes, and tables, respectively.

B

D

P

R

S

T